YOUR THIRD BRAIN

The Revolutionary New Discovery
to Achieve Optimum Health

YOUR THIRD BRAIN: THE REVOLUTIONARY NEW DISCOVERY TO ACHIEVE OPTIMUM HEALTH

by Peter Greenlaw and Marco Ruggiero MD with Drew Greenlaw

ISBN: 978-0-9882771-4-4

© Peter Greenlaw, 2015

Printed in the United States of America

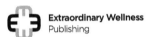 Extraordinary Wellness
Publishing

Extraordinary Wellness Publishing

#235-6834 South University Blvd

Centennial, CO 80122

The New Health Conversation Series

DISCLAIMER: None of the following statements in this book have been evaluated by the FDA. This book is for educational purposes only. This book was written to make you aware of what is available. It is up to you to decide if this information can help you to maximize your wellness potential. It is always recommended to consult with your medical doctor or health professional before embarking on any new diet, nutritional protocol, or exercise regimen.

TABLE OF CONTENTS

Chapter 4. Exciting Published Observational Studies 91

Chapter 5. Evaluating a Patient's Health 109

SECTION II

Chapter 9. The Microbiome Protocol and Regimen............... 173

Chapter 10. Mysteries of Wonder Molecules
from Heparin to GcMAF 213

Chapter 11. The Use of Ultrasound for the Third Brain 231

ACKNOWLEDGMENTS

First and foremost, I want to thank Marco Ruggiero, MD and his wife Stefania Pacini, MD. They are two of the most brilliant medical doctors and researchers on the planet. I am grateful to them for introducing my son and me to their amazing research. This book is in great part the story of their brilliant discoveries, which are already having a significant impact on the world.

Next, thank you to my amazing book-coaching and marketing team led by Melissa G Wilson of Networlding, who is helping me to change the world.

I also want to thank Michelle Kriegel for her time, invaluable editing, and input that helped bring *Your Third Brain* to a completely new level. Also, a big thank you to T.L. Price, our brilliant book layout person. This book truly would not exist if it were not for her tireless dedication.

I also want to add thanks to Bob Sievewright for his encouragement and valuable insights on this book.

Thanks to my great friend Doug Freel, my amazing director and co-producer for having the vision and confidence to create our upcoming Television Series: *What if You Didn't Know?*

Special thanks to Dylan Garity for the final edits and his devotion to getting it right.

I cannot express how proud and thankful to our coauthor, my oldest son, Drew Greenlaw, graduate of the University of Colorado School of Journalism, for his sleepless nights and hours and hours of research to bring this amazing story to life.

To my wonderful wife Sarah and my youngest son Colin, who have now seen dreams come true for our family.

Finally, thank you John for your amazing belief and trust in me more than a decade ago. You told me to go forward with the research when I did not believe I could do it. Thank you from the bottom of my heart. You are responsible for so much of my success.

FOREWORD

Ten years after I published *Men Are from Mars, Women Are from Venus*, I suddenly realized that there was more to making relationships better than new communication skills. Optimum brain function was also just as important.

It is not possible to sustain intimacy and happiness in a relationship if we are stressed, tired, anxious, and unable to enjoy our lives. If the brain is not supported with good nutrition, love alone is not enough. This insight set me on a new path.

This journey began when I was diagnosed with early-stage Parkinson's disease. After getting the diagnosis, I immediately focused my time, energy and resources on finding a natural solution. After six months of healing my brain, I not only recovered, but also felt even better than before. By supporting my brain function with natural supplements and nutrients, I discovered how much easier a relationship can be. With a sustained positive mood and plenty of energy and motivation, my relationships with my wife and family improved. I couldn't wait to share my discoveries.

I opened a wellness center to teach what I had learned. For ten years, with the help of many health researchers and experts, I continued my exploration while also educating thousands of individuals, couples and families about optimal nutrition for better relationships and optimal brain health. Over the last decade, I wrote a series of books revealing many of these insights.

After making a few dietary changes and adding good nutrition, I witnessed individuals, couples and families experience profound transformations. This experience was very rewarding, but the results were not always the same. Most would experience dramatic positive changes within days, but not all. Something was missing, but I kept searching.

Two years ago, while updating my research into natural solutions for cancer, I came across a growing body of medical research on a particular protein called GcMAF. It was helping cancer patients by activating vitamin D and strengthening the immune system. I was further intrigued to discover that this same protein was also helping people with chronic fatigue, and even children with autism.

I had to try it and share it with all my friends and family. Although I was quite healthy, after trying it, I still experienced a burst of new energy and greater clarity. My friends with digestive issues had immediate improvement as well as greater energy and clarity. Combining a natural form of GcMAF with my other suggestions for optimal brain function was having even more profound results than my previous protocols.

Although I have written several books on the subject of stress, hormones and optimal brain performance, this vital information was missing. It is new and has been unavailable until now… that is, until this book, *Your Third Brain*.

This revolutionary book provides the missing insight to fully understand how to develop your life potential. Understanding the existence of the third brain is possibly the most exciting discovery of the last century. The natural production of the special protein GcMAF is but one of the many benefits of understanding and supporting the third brain. That is why I was honored and pleased to write the foreword for this amazing new book by Peter Greenlaw, Marco Ruggiero MD and Drew Greenlaw.

It has now been more than a decade since I met Peter. When we first met, he told me about his two sons, Drew and Colin. Colin, his youngest son, had real challenges with concentration and anxiety, and had been given prescription drugs to deal with his issues.

Fortunately I was able to give Peter and Colin my research on natural alternatives that have worked for thousands of my clients. Within a week, Colin did extremely well using the all-natural solutions.

Peter became fascinated with my research and I, along with many other experts, have mentored him over the last decade. He is a huge supporter of my research and has introduced it to more than 1,000 audiences worldwide.

A year ago, in 2014, Peter was asked to be a speaker at Autism One in Chicago, one of the largest autism conferences in the world. Peter had called and asked me if I had any research on Autism that I might share with him. At my wellness center, we had been getting great results with autistic children. He flew out to my home in California and I shared my research, including new breakthrough research on Autism by an Italian doctor, Marco Ruggiero MD.

Dr. Ruggiero was also the keynote speaker at Autism One. I feel a great pride in being responsible for Peter meeting Dr. Ruggiero at the Autism One Conference. That meeting resulted in the joint collaboration on this wonderful new book, *Your Third Brain*.

Your Third Brain is truly going to change the way we look at everything, as it relates to maximizing our quality of life and our wellness potential.

Almost 20 years ago, scientists and researchers had discovered that we in fact had a second brain. This second brain, which contains as many neurons as in the first brain, was discovered in our gut (Gastrointestinal Tract). The discovery of this second brain has led to a change in the way that psychological conditions are now being approached. Many in psychiatry are treating mental challenges first in the gut with remarkable success.

For many adults and children, simply giving up the hard-to-digest gluten in wheat products or casein in pasteurized milk products has dramatically relieved the symptoms of ADHD to Parkinson's. This was truly a huge discovery.

This discovery of the second brain has now been overshadowed by a major new discovery made just 4 ½ years ago, a discovery that should give us all renewed hope that we can, through science, greatly improve the quality of our lives from a health and wellness potential point of view.

In my research, I have seen a lot of breakthroughs, but I have never encountered such an amazing scientific discovery. You, of course, can judge for yourself.

This discovery of the "Third Brain" by Dr. Ruggiero was not only amazing for its groundbreaking scientific implications, but also for me personally. My friends, family, clients and staff are all thanking me for introducing them to *Your Third Brain* with its unique protocols and regimens.

Your Third Brain lays out how Marco Ruggiero, MD/PhD in molecular biology, realized that an organ (the microbiome) that had gone undetected in human anatomy for nearly 3000 years was in fact a third brain and not just another organ.

In this book, Dr. Ruggiero, Peter Greenlaw and his son Drew tell the story of the third brain. They lay out in intimate detail not only this amazing discovery, but most importantly go into what this great discovery can mean for a higher quality of life for all of us.

In just over 4 ½ years since the discovery of the third brain (the scientific name is the microbiome), Dr. Ruggiero and his colleagues have published observational studies in some of some of the most prestigious medical journals in the world.

These observational studies are very promising for supporting our immune system, cardiovascular support, optimal brain function, and graceful aging. It goes without saying that ongoing research is needed and will be done.

Many of the published studies utilized a probiotic super food created by Dr. Ruggiero and his wife Stefania Pacini MD. After years of research, Ruggiero and Pacini's hard work paid off, and they were finally able to discover and create a super food for the third brain.

This is a food that uses the same fermentation process that is created at our birth. Dr. Ruggiero and his wife Stefania Pacini used all of their combined years of scientific knowledge in molecular biology, anatomy, and nutritional science to successfully reverse engineer the combination of fungi, bacteria, yeast and microbes picked up by the baby through the birth process.

Then they figured out that the fermentation process and interaction of colostrum (the clear liquid created before breast milk) and mother's breast milk with the bacteria, fungi, yeast and microbes begins the process to create the third brain (the microbiome).

Thomas Edison once said that he had not failed 3,000 times in inventing the lightbulb, that instead, he had figured out 3,000 ways not to invent the lightbulb.

In a very similar way, Dr. Ruggiero and Stefania also figured out, through thousands of hours and attempts and sleepless nights, how not to invent this super food. Then, finally, they figured out the successful formula, and the super food for the third brain was a reality.

This super food for the third brain has now been used by thousands of individuals, including healthy individuals like me as well as those with health challenges. This book also lays out the best foods for the "first brain" in our heads, as well as the optimum foods for our second brain in the gut.

The main goal of Dr. Ruggiero and Dr. Pacini is to give people the possibility of a high quality of life for as long as possible. It has been such a pleasure for me to meet, learn from and interact with Dr. Ruggiero and Dr. Pacini. It is truly a great gift they have provided for the world.

I am excited for you to read *Your Third Brain* and discover, as I did, what is now available for all of you. This is truly a book everyone should read as soon as they can get their hands on it.

Dr. John Gray

PREFACE

As I sit here at 34,000 feet flying across the country, I think about the marvel of man's ingenuity that has led to many world-changing discoveries. I gaze out the window of this amazing machine. Here I am, flying, not with clouds between my knees, but with them out my window, as we soar. The Wright Brothers certainly believed the impossible was possible, literally flying with clouds between *their* knees.

We have become so accustomed to life-changing, almost magical inventions that we often take their innovations for granted. We turn a switch and a room is no longer dark. We press a few buttons and we are able to get from point A to point B in our cars. Doctors are able to remove organs by only making a tiny slit in our bodies. We have immunizations for many of the most dreadful diseases, and the pharmaceutical industry has come quite far in finding drugs and vaccines for many of these ailments. The trend has been to find cures using a pill or shot.

We call this *procedural intervention* as opposed to what we think should be more widely used and that is *preventive intervention*. We have the best doctors, surgeons and prescription drugs (procedural interventions) in the world. The United States spends nearly 2 ½ times more on healthcare than any of the other industrialized countries in the world, and yet the U.S. most recently ranked 50th in life expectancy.[1]

We have come so far in certain areas of medicine, yet still have not scratched the surface when it comes to maximizing our wellness potential. With such a surge of technology and advancement, sometimes innovation is right in front of us. Maybe it has been around for several decades, and we just haven't completely realized its amazing potential.

Is it so hard to believe that there are still many, many things we can learn from the mysteries of nature? Doctors and scientists no longer question the electricity that powers their operating rooms and miraculous medical devices that, when first presented, seemed like magic.

I have asked this question before—is this group of medical doctors and researchers any different from those people a few hundred years ago who stuck to their belief that the world was flat? I certainly hope that the attitudes are now beginning to change.

The HBO documentary *Escape Fire* warned us that we very well might be witnessing the first signs of the collapse of our current health-care system due to the fact that it relies principally on

---

1. https://www.cia.gov/library/publications/the-world-factbook/rankorder/2102rank.html

the concept of procedural intervention. The overwhelming use of procedural intervention may also be in large part due to the fact that there is almost no compensation for preventative interventional approaches. We pointed this out in our book, *The TDOS Syndrome and Solutions*. Doctors are compensated disproportionately, for how many procedures they perform instead of on how well they handle preventative advice.

These great doctors and scientists are hopefully becoming more open to and aware of preventative interventional approaches in conjunction with traditional medical approaches. This was very apparent to me when I attended an integrated medical conference called *Science and Connection: A New Era of Integrative Health and Medicine*.

In just one year, this conference increased its attendance by nearly 200 percent. This five-day conference was both educational and inspirational. Speaker after speaker emphasized that as medical doctors, they must explore and integrate into their practices the published results of preventative approaches with their patients. They feel this is a new era in medicine and that by combining all their medical training and procedural interventions, there is new hope for the future.

This approach of combining preventative interventional approaches with traditional medicine may lengthen the quality of life even for those with the most severe health challenges. With such a surge of technology and advancement, sometimes innovation is right in front of us. Maybe it has been around for several decades. We just haven't seen or realized its true potential.

Why is it that many continue to ignore what is a growing, grassroots style of medicine (preventative interventional approaches)? In particular, one of the most promising and now highly researched preventative interventional approaches, called "immunotherapy", has been practiced for over 100 years. This involves healing the body by supporting and empowering the immune system.

Many holistic, medical, and allopathic practitioners are taking a serious look at this immunotherapeutic approach of prevention and natural healing. The doctors and researchers are greatly encouraged by what they have observed and have thus published in peer-reviewed medical journals. We are hoping that more Western-style practitioners become aware of immunotherapeutic intervention's positive effects on their patients and, in turn, make it a larger part of their practices. Moreover, we hope that you, as a reader, will become aware of its preventive potential and how it can let you take more control of your wellness and thus its potentially positive outcomes.

The premise of *Your Third Brain* is to take a complex look inside the human body and to learn how we can be proactive in our ability to maximize our wellness potential and our quality of life. It's that simple.

THE RESULT

The impossible may, in fact, become an everyday occurrence. In this book, co-author Marco Ruggiero, MD and PhD of Molecular Biology, modern-day pioneer and crusader, has already demonstrated great courage in the face of threats of imprisonment because of his research. Despite these threats, he will share this research and the discoveries he has made with you. His work is so important that it may one day prove to be one of the answers in assisting the body in healing itself and living healthier longer.

Thank goodness Dr. Ruggiero did not waiver in the face of such threats to his personal freedom. He had a burning desire and belief to change the world through what he and his colleagues were discovering in the laboratory. These discoveries took years and have been scientifically validated in more than 150 published papers in major peer-reviewed journals.

Additionally, a large number of medical doctors are now utilizing Dr. Ruggiero's research and discoveries alongside conventional medical approaches, producing very promising outcomes for their patients. The work of this brave doctor and his colleagues is ongoing and offers incredible hope for the future. Our intentions for this book are to introduce the discovery of the three brains and their interconnectivity to our overall health and wellness. In the short span of the past ten years, scientists have discovered that we have a second brain in addition to the brain that resides inside our skull.

THE SECOND BRAIN

The second brain is your gut, formally known as the gastrointestinal tract. It has as many neurotransmitters as the first brain (in our heads). In fact, many psychiatrists are now treating patients with psychological challenges by first addressing problems in the gut.

Four and a half years ago, a huge discovery was made. We call this discovery "the third brain". In 2010, a team of researchers discovered a new organ that had gone undetected for more than 3,000 years in Human Anatomy. They called this newly discovered organ the microbiome.

Although Dr. Ruggiero did not discover the microbiome, he did identify it as *The Third Brain*. We will go into great detail as to why the third brain should give mankind such hope to maximize everyone's wellness potential.

For example, imagine if anatomists had not yet identified the heart and you had chest pains, numbness in your arm, or suddenly could not breathe? When the EMTs arrive, how could they possibly begin to treat you?

The microbiome is made up of bacteria, viruses, fungi, yeast and microbes. About seventy percent of the microbiome is contained in the lining of the GI Tract; the other thirty percent is dispersed in our mucosa, skin, blood, hair and throughout the rest of the body. If we analyze this, it means that we are less than 1% human as to the number of genes that are part of our human being, and the other more than 99% of our genes are microbial.

WE LIVE IN THE THIRD BRAIN'S ECOSYSTEM

Now imagine, by making the world aware of the third brain, what is possible. For more than 3,000 years, anatomists were unaware of the presence of this organ. It essentially means that a good number of medical practitioners have been focusing all of their attention on just 1% of us. They have done a miraculous job with the information they have had to work with.

Now visualize the medical world being introduced to the third brain and the possibility to interact with the other 99% of the human body. This is a game-changing discovery. This is the story of the life-changing work of Dr. Marco Ruggiero with his wife, Dr. Stefania

Pacini, and their team of researchers. Their amazing interactions since 2011 with the third brain will leave you speechless. Their team of researchers are bringing hope and excitement to thousands of people with health challenges as a way of maximizing their quality of life.

Dr. Ruggiero's team are also working hand in hand with the complete cooperation and unprecedented collaboration of medical doctors, with the goal of extending the highest possible quality of life for their patients for as long as possible. To this end, they have published many papers about their work in prestigious peer-reviewed medical journals. It is important to point out that this successful formula is a combination of the most advanced medical procedures in combination with the interactions, approaches and regimens that Dr. Ruggiero and his team have discovered in the scientifically demonstrated healing support of the third brain.

This ongoing scientific quest has far-reaching potential for all of us, not just for patients facing health challenges. These scientific discoveries also seem to indicate this newly discovered healing potential of our third brain. Understanding the third brain and how it works can give all of us the best support for our immune systems. And that, in and of itself, may be the best preventative interventional strategy to work with and enhance the science of conventional medicine.

Our goal in this book is to make you aware of what is available today. Our goal is also to educate you on the technologies and protocols that have been designed to maximize wellness.

It is our honor and privilege to introduce you to this hero, astounding colleague, and friend, Dr. Marco Ruggiero. This book is devoted to making the world aware of Dr. Ruggiero's groundbreaking research and discoveries.

We hope this book will enlighten your perception of what is available in "The New Health Conversation™".

Sincerely,

Peter Greenlaw

November, 2014

NOTE: *Your Third Brain* is not a cure for any disease or chronic illness. This book is about making the world aware of specific protocols and regimens that, in combination with conventional medical science, may extend the quality of life for all of us.

Preventative interventional or alternative (holistic approaches) do not work as a substitute for traditional medicine, drugs or medical interventions. It is always recommended you check with your doctor or health professional before embarking on any diet or preventative interventional approach.

None of these statements have been evaluated by the Food and Drug Administration. This book is not intended to treat or diagnose any disease. The information contained in this book is from the work of Dr. Marco Ruggiero, which has been published in over 150 peer reviewed scientific journals. It is always recommended to check with your doctor before embarking on any new health care protocol.

1

Marco's Story and the Importance of This Book

Following are excerpts from an interview that I conducted with Dr. Marco Ruggiero over the summer of 2014. I was instantly fascinated with his research and the career path he chose to follow. To me, Marco is a pioneer, pushing the limits of what we think we know. Time and time again, Dr. Ruggiero has pushed the limit of what the scientific community has deemed the norm. By doing this, Dr. Ruggiero has made major breakthroughs in preventative medicine and has discovered secrets of the body that have gone undetected for over a century.

MARCO: I was born in Firenze, Italy, in 1956. I hold a PhD in Molecular Biology.

I am a certified Medical Doctor specializing in Clinical Radiology, and I am a full professor of Molecular Biology at the Department of Experimental and Clinical Biomedical Sciences of the University of Firenze, Italy. I served in the army as a Medical Lieutenant with specific training in chemical, biological, and nuclear warfare.

I worked at Burroughs Wellcome Company in North Carolina, where I published a seminal paper with Nobel Laureate Sir John Vane. I later worked at the National Cancer Institute of the NIH in Bethesda, with Dr. Stuart A. Aaronson and Dr. Peter Duesberg. Since 1992 I have held the chair of Molecular Biology at the University of Firenze, where I lead a research group of about 10 researchers. I have been published in more than 150 peer-reviewed scientific papers. But let me back up a little bit.

In the year of my birth, Soviet tanks invaded Hungary and massacred people who sought freedom from Communist oppression. I grew up during the worst of the Cold War, knowing my country could be invaded at any time. I developed a fighting, rebellious spirit, which has been with me all my life, and which has formed my scientific and academic career.

I earned my MD from the University of Firenze in 1980. Soon after that, I entered the military. While I cut my teeth on atomic, biological, and chemical warfare, I was eventually sent to Houston at the end of 1982.

There, my task was to gather information on an emerging epidemic, which was thought somehow to be connected to chemical or biological warfare. It turns out that it was completely unrelated.

After leaving the military, I spent two years at the Department of Molecular Biology of Burroughs Wellcome Company in the Research Triangle Park of North Carolina, working on intracellular signal transduction and protease inhibitors, which, simply put, are a class of molecules and their structures.

There, I had the opportunity to meet Sir John Vane, a genius who was awarded the Nobel Prize in Physiology and Medicine in 1982. Sir John Vane was so impressed by my research that, being himself a prominent member of the Academy of Sciences of the USA, he sponsored a paper of mine for publication in the Proceedings of the Academy.

After my postdoctoral period at Burroughs Wellcome Co., I moved to the National Cancer Institute (NCI) of the National Institutes of Health in Bethesda, where I worked for several years in the Laboratory of Cellular and Molecular Biology under the direction of Dr. Stuart A. Aaronson.

There, I was fortunate enough to share an office with Professor Peter Duesberg, often termed "the world's most reviled genius," who was on sabbatical from Berkeley. We became friends. Our intellectual and scientific collaboration produced significant achievements regarding the importance of the human immune system. My central point was (and is) very simple: given years of failures in fighting viruses, the scientific community must change its focus away from the virus and to the immune system itself.

Let's restore the immune system and allow the restored immune system to take care of the virus. For us, all this was very logical and very simple: let's rebuild the immune system, and the immune system will get rid of the virus, without the need to prescribe toxic drugs.

In other words, an empowered immune system can help eradicate infection and viruses without the need to use antiviral drugs with all their side effects.

PETER: Before we go further into your background, what motivated you? What drove you to work on ideas that everyone else told you were impossible? I see you as a modern-day Christopher Columbus. When the smartest people in the world told him the world was flat, Columbus sailed off regardless of what the "experts" thought… What drove you? What motivated you to bypass what others said was impossible in order to clear that uncharted path?

DR. RUGGIERO: They are still saying it! I think it is two things. First of all, whether it is true or not, it is said in my family that Giuseppe Garibaldi, the famous hero of the two world wars (The Austro-Prussian War, and the Third Italian War of Independence) was my ancestor. I know that he had a relationship with an ancestor of my grandfather, but I don't know whether I have genes of this revolutionary hero of the past or not. So I don't know whether it is genetic or not. But what really drove me was not to go against the prevailing dogma. I think it was something simpler: curiosity. Cancer, as well as autism, neurodegenerative disease and all of these diseases that still remain kind of a mystery today, they evoke a great curiosity. I am a very curious person. It is my nature. I don't think I have any merit for this. I am just naturally curious. Since I was educated as a medical doctor and a researcher, I am very curious to find out the basic mechanisms that make cancer cells so proficient. Why are they so efficient, and what makes them so fast-growing?

What makes them invisible to the immune system surveillance when the immune system should control them, yet evidently fails? From there, I wanted to provide relief for the sufferers of these diseases. I never forgot my time being a medical doctor, even after all my days, months and years spent at the lab bench, far away from the bedside. Eventually, I wanted to provide some result that could bring relief, some hope or some treatment to people who are suffering from cancer, not just to publish a paper for *Science*. I don't know if this answers your question, but I think if you wanted to summarize in one single word what is *still* driving me, even though I am 58 now (I am not so young anymore), it's curiosity. I am curious.

PETER: I understand that to become a medical doctor is quite an undertaking. And you also have a PhD in molecular biology? What came first? What drove you to further your education?

DR. RUGGIERO: Yes, exactly. This revelation came when I was in the army. That was 1982 to '83.

PETER: Now, were you already a medical doctor then?

DR. RUGGIERO: Yes, I was a medical doctor. I was a lieutenant medical officer. And since I could speak a little bit of English in those days, and since I had a little bit of culture, the high command sent me to the United States. They sent me here in 1982. They asked me to conduct and expand on some ideas I had at the time. So I came here; I gathered information; I learned many things, some of which I wish I had not learned, because they changed my perspective. At the same time, I became truly infatuated with research. I realized that all I had learned in my years of medical school was plenty, if I wished to cure patients. But that was not enough for me.

So I became enamored with research, with biological research. That's why after having finished the military, I decided to enter into research in molecular biology. I chose molecular biology because it is a field where you are still working with living things, cells, biology, but at the molecular level. That is at the most intimate level, where things happen. So you are not a chemist, you are a biologist; you are still a medical doctor if you wish, but you are working with the most intimate mechanisms that regulate the life and death of our cells, and therefore the life and death of our bodies. So that's exactly when, if you asked me, this love of research arose. It was in those years in the military. So I have to thank the military for this as well.

PETER: You are working on something that could change the world. Isn't it ironic that some of the answers may lie within us, not outside us? Isn't that amazing? We're talking on the molecular level—and at this molecular level, we can possibly establish our true wellness potential?

DR. RUGGIERO: Absolutely. Yes. From the molecular point of view, when we are born, we already have cancer cells in our body. All of us have cancer cells at any age of our life. This is because mutations happen randomly and also because pollution in our environment increases the probability of mutations. Luckily, we do not develop cancer when we are newborns, and we do not develop cancer until we are relatively old, usually in the fifth decade of our life. Why is that, if we have cancer cells throughout our lives? Because our immune system is able to recognize these cancer cells as aberrant mutant cells and destroy them. Mainly, this is due to a particular type of cells that are called macrophages. The word 'macrophage' derives from Greek: 'macro' means big, 'phage' means eater. So, 'big eater.' Actually they do recognize cancer cells, cells infected by viruses, or cells that have been corrupted for whatever reason. They recognize them as a danger for the body, and they attach to them and truly eat them.

PETER: Like the video and arcade game Pac Man?

DR. RUGGIERO: Truly, like Pac Man. We have pictures, shot in our lab, where we can see activated macrophages eat. They deconstruct, and they *destroy*, the cancer cells. This happens on a daily basis. This is happening in our bodies right now. When this does not happen, because the macrophages are weak, or because they are kind of blind (like sentinels), or they are not well fed, or they do not have the proper tools to identify the enemy, possibly from a distance, then the cancer cells can multiply. And from one they become two, and then there is exponential growth. At that point, the enemy inside is too big to be destroyed by the few macrophages that we have.

PETER: I know you've been working on this for more than 30 years. When did it occur to you that what you were doing was really going to make a difference? Along with what you have learned as a medical doctor, with radiation therapy and chemotherapy, etc., how did you come to the conclusion that there could be something else that could help make those two primary treatments, for cancer in this case, more effective? When did you realize that by employing the immune system along with the other primary treatments that your arsenal to heal became more effective? When did you think this was worthy of your time and effort? You've devoted three decades to it, so there must have been a point when you thought it was worth it, more than just curiosity. I know you still work very hard, very long hours with patients and with your research. When was it that the light went on and you knew you were on the right track? Maybe you hadn't discovered it yet. Maybe you hadn't seen the outcome, but there was a point when you exclaimed that "this is my life's work, my dream." When did that occur?

DR. RUGGIERO: My dream was very clear. It was to find some further treatment for cancer. There are treatments out there that are very efficient. They provide a lot of benefits. Today, many types of cancer that were deadly only a few decades ago can be treated. But still, it is not enough. So if you ask me, *when* I developed the willingness to transfer my research from the bench to the bedside was actually in October of 1984. I had just moved to Chapel Hill, NC, to live for a few months. When I left my family in August, everything was going well. After a couple of months, I received a telephone call, where, with proper words, they didn't quite know how to tell me, they had discovered that my father had stage IV cancer. It was completely out of the blue. When I left, he had been completely healthy. But he had stage IV cancer of the throat with metastasis in his neck lymph nodes.

At that point I decided, okay, it's nice to be here, to publish papers and advance my academic career, but I want to do something for my father, first, and then for all cancer patients. My father died in 2006. He died of old age 22 years after his diagnosis. With him, we succeeded. But that was not enough for me, and from that very day, I began to work in both realms. From the lab, I began looking at molecules, tiny molecules that have absurd or unpronounceable names. I wrote several papers, one on the molecule phosphatidylinositol 4,5-bisphosphate, but from researching these tiny molecules, I never forgot that my aim was not only to study molecular mechanisms just to satisfy an intellectual curiosity, but to find a way to provide some sort of relief or benefit to people like my father. And, if you ask me when exactly I decided to move from the bench to the bedside, that happened in 2010, more or less. We were observing stage IV cancer patients at the time. As you know, stage IV cancer is the end. It's when the patient is labeled incurable, inoperable and untreatable. Essentially, patients are told, "Listen, we have done everything we can at this point. Now, go home and put your things in order, because there is nothing else we can do for you." So we were dealing specifically with this type of cancer patient.

PETER: Terminally ill cancer patients?

DR. RUGGIERO: Yes, the incurable, hopeless cancer patients. We observed that some people actually died within a few weeks of their diagnosis, while other people lived much longer. We began to investigate what was happening. Why were some people with the same stage of cancer, the same age, all with similar conditions, living only a few weeks and others up to four or five years? In oncology, if you survive more than five years from the initial diagnosis, then you are considered cured. What happens the next day is irrelevant from a statistical point of view. But the follow-up is for five years. So we could say the term, 'cure for cancer' is kind of a slippery statement. We should say that if you survive more than five years, you can consider yourself somewhat cured.

So, how did this come about? We noticed that the key difference was nutrition and the immune system. In other words, those who had poor nutrition and a poorly working immune system died within a few weeks. From the nutritional point of view, I must tell you, in Europe it is the same as it is in the United States, and most people are malnourished. Usually, when we talk about malnutrition, we think about skinny boys in Africa. That's a type of malnutrition. But also, malnutrition is when you do not have the proper balance between the macronutrients, which are carbohydrates or sugars, proteins, and lipids. When you have the wrong ratio of these three macronutrients, you can talk about malnutrition.

So people here, just like in Europe, are malnourished. Malnutrition brings about a number of other problems to our body, because it unbalances all the equilibrium in our body. Again, looking at these stage IV cancer patients, all of them had undergone surgery, chemotherapy as well as radiation therapy and were left hopeless. There was nothing they could do. Now, those who had malnutrition and poor immune systems, they lived only six months on average. But those for whom we were able to implement a program of proper nutrition with high proteins, nutrients, minerals, and anti-inflammatory fats, and to boost the immune system, the average survival was four years. And we published this in 2012 in the *American Journal of Immunology* in cooperation with colleagues from Germany and other hospitals in Italy, so it's not only our research group. It's been out in the public domain since 2012. At that time, we were not working on any specific molecule that was activating the immune system.

We only focused on nutrition, and we were able to change the prognosis of a terminally ill cancer patient from six months to four years, which is not bad, especially considering that those who lived for four years had once been labeled as doomed to die within a few weeks. And they lived four years, with excellent quality of life. So this has been published, and this is only one paper out of the many that have the same basic information. Nutrition is the basis for every treatment. Every treatment for every chronic condition, from cancer to autism to Alzheimer's to Parkinson's, if it (the treatment) is not grounded in proper nutrition, is doomed to fail, or not to be as efficient as it could be. So the potential for any specific treatment for any specific condition lies with nutrition. If your nutrition is not properly adapted to your condition, then you cannot explain the big results from any type of drug or treatment.

PETER: So identifying a lack of proper nutrition and a weak immune system when attacking disease was a major breakthrough in your research? I also think your "Eureka moment" occurred when you began to identify what was happening on a cellular and molecular level.

DR. RUGGIERO: As researchers, we rarely have those eureka moments. Instead, insights come after hours and hours and years and years at the bench with frustrating experiments that we cannot reproduce. Most of the time, the eureka moment is retrospective. That is, after 30 years of research, you look back and you think that you have found something.

PETER: So like Thomas Edison said, "I didn't fail 3,000 times inventing the lightbulb, I just found 3,000 ways not to invent the lightbulb".

DR. RUGGIERO: Oh yes, most of our experiments are failures. But failure means that we have a hypothesis and we have results that are sometimes the complete opposite of what the hypothesis was. But, we learn because those are not failures. Nature does not obey our hypotheses. It's we who have to learn from nature. So we observe how nature works at the molecular, cellular, or organism level. So after 30-some years, we came up with a combination of approaches that we felt confident bringing to the patient. That's why we developed what we call the protocols. These protocols target the underlying molecular mechanisms, which are responsible not only for the onset but also for the progression of these diseases. Now I will mention only two, cancer and autism, because those are the two diseases where we have anecdotal evidence that we can target some if not all chronic diseases, because we went back to this allgemeine pathology concept. We are not targeting the final symptom. We are not lowering the fever with aspirin. Rather, we are trying to *eliminate* the cause of the fever.

PETER: So the other way to say that is that you're not fighting the fires, you're trying to find out what caused the fire.

DR. RUGGIERO: You can translate it in English as "general pathology," but it is more than that. The German scientists, a hundred and some years ago, had a very clear intuition. That is, diseases show up with different symptoms. You can have infectious diseases, inflammation, cancer, neurodegenerative diseases, and a thousand other diseases.

But the core alterations were the same for all diseases. In other words, cancer, infectious diseases and neurodegenerative diseases at the cellular level, at the molecular level, shared common features. This is what *allgemeine* in German means. That is, something that comprises all, which, translated from Italian is general pathology, but 'general' doesn't give the full idea. In any case, I was fascinated by this concept, that although diseases appear with different symptoms and affect an array of people at different ages of life, nevertheless, if you get down to the basic level, the cellular or molecular level, the alterations are all the same. The reasoning went that if you understood those alterations, then you had tools with which to restore the original balance, the original homeostasis as we say, or equilibrium, so that essentially with a few tools you could deal with a number of different diseases.

Now, some 40 years later, this is exactly what I am trying to do with the molecules we are working with today. Cancer and other chronic diseases that have their roots in the mutations within the human body (which are in turn caused by damage induced from the environment and through modern lifestyles) are extremely complex and individual issues. We cannot say something is valid for all patients or diagnoses. I have been working in the field of immunotherapy for almost three decades, and I am happy to say that some forms of chemotherapy and surgery can be useful. There are patients who will never undergo chemotherapy because they do not wish to trade the effects of the toxic therapy for two to three more months of life. It's up to the individual patient and his or her physician to decide on the best course.

PETER: Thank you for you for our great work and devotion to finding the answers to the impossible.

This book and the approach to rebalance the body in order to support and empower the immune system is Dr. Ruggiero's novel approach to combating many of the health challenges we face today. It is a method that uses the human body as its ally rather than bludgeoning the body with chemicals and radiation in order to hammer it into submission. We are in no way replacing, eliminating or substituting the use of conventional medical approaches. Instead, we are working with them to hopefully improve the quality of everyone's life.

EMPOWERING THE BODY'S SOLDIERS

We empower the body's soldiers rather than lay waste to all on the battlefield. We approach the body as a total being, rather than isolate faulty mechanisms and attempt to rip them out.

If this approach makes sense to you and, more importantly, if it gives you hope, then read on. It will challenge you. It is a paradigm shift, and as always happens when an old paradigm is abandoned and a new one proposed, we must change our point of view if we are to succeed. This is a success worth embracing.

2

The First and Second Brain

It's no secret that for centuries, humans have explored the human mind, searching for life's mysteries regarding how the brain worked and how it managed to control the rest of the body. The brain in our skull, the one we are all familiar with, has always been deemed as the body's headquarters (pun intended). It is perceived as grand central station, management, etc. It also seemed to play a prominent role in everything we see as being human, from language to emotions and beyond. The first brain is what we thought separated us from the rest of the living creatures roaming the planet.

It is common knowledge that the brain is an organ of the body in the head that controls functions, movements, sensations and thoughts. Although the structure of the first brain is similar between humans and mammals, the cerebral cortex of the human brain is developed greater than that of any other mammal. This chapter is not arguing with the function or importance of the brain we are all so familiar with. With all the advanced technology in this day and age, it has come to light that there is more than one manager in the body. It actually makes some sense when you think about the miracle of the human body and everything that it encompasses.

The information in this book and this chapter is not speculation. It is a fact that the brain has a second and third brain to assist the body with all of its functions. Not all thought and emotion starts in the first brain. The importance of these discoveries is changing the role of medicine, food, allergies, illnesses, etc. for civilization. There will be a time when it seemed silly to think that humans believed there was only one functioning brain. In fact, humans at one time thought it hilarious that the world was round. A medical breakthrough of this magnitude will help change and mold the world for all future generations.

DISCOVERY OF A SECOND BRAIN

The concept of a second brain emerged several years ago with the discovery of neurons that are embedded in the walls of the GI tract. In addition to these neurons, there are other cells that are designated interstitial cells of Cajal, named after Santiago Ramón y Cajal, a Spanish pathologist, histologist, neuroscientist, and Nobel laureate. These cells are found intertwined among neurons embedded within the smooth muscles lining the gut. According to the early studies of Cajal, these cells served as the generator and pacemaker of the slow waves of contraction that move material along the GI tract, thus mediating neurotransmission from motor nerves to smooth muscle cells. In other words, in the days of Cajal, at the turn of the nineteenth century, it was hypothesized that the neurons in the GI tract only served to move the products of digestion through the intestine and that they were subjugated to the influence of the brain that it is inside our heads.

It has been known for some time that mood influences the function of the GI tract. Many people suffer stomach distress when they are anxious or stressed. However, until recently, it was only hypothesized that the GI tract simply responded, in a sort of a passive way, to the inputs that came from inside our heads. The neurons of the GI tract were considered mere executors of the orders that came from above, with no ability whatsoever to generate anything that could be defined as "thought" or "emotions".

After the pioneering work of Cajal, it was discovered that in the GI tract, there are about one hundred million neurons. That is one thousandth of the number of neurons in the brain inside our heads, and essentially the same number of neurons as are in the spinal cord. Therefore, the concept of a "second brain" embedded in the walls of our GI tract, began to emerge. In fact, those neurons not only are interconnected with each other, but they are also interconnected with the neurons inside our heads and, after decades of neglect, it was hypothesized that their role could go well beyond that of simply "obeying" the orders that came from above. In other words, in the past decade, it has been first hypothesized and then demonstrated that the flux of information within the body is not unidirectional, from the head to the gut, but bi-directional, and the neurons in the GI tract influence the behavior of those in the brain and vice-versa.

It was the discovery of the complexity of these neural networks that led to the concept of the second brain. It should be said, however, that the denomination "second brain" might not be anatomically correct. In fact, in all pair organs, we do not describe them as first and second; instead, we talk of left and right kidneys or lungs. As far as the brains (plural) are concerned, we should envision the neurons in the GI tract, the so-called "second brain" (simply because it was discovered millennia after the first one) just as another anatomical part of the brain. In other words, we should describe the second brain simply as another anatomical part of the brain, just like the frontal or parietal lobes or the cerebellum. And just like those other parts of the brain inside our heads, the second brain can operate autonomously or in conjunction with the other parts of the brain.

It normally communicates with the neurons inside our heads through the vagus nerve and sympathetic system, and for these communications, it makes use of more than 30 neurotransmitters, most of which are identical to the ones found in the neurons inside our heads, such as acetylcholine, dopamine, and serotonin. Oddly enough, more than 90% of the body's serotonin lies in the gut, as well as about 50% of the body's dopamine, which is currently being studied to further our understanding of its function in the brain. There are further similarities with the brain inside our heads; there are cells that are similar to the astroglia of the brain, a sort of connective tissue, and a diffusion barrier around the capillaries surrounding ganglia that is similar to the blood brain barrier of cerebral blood vessels.

With the increase in knowledge about the anatomy and the physiology of the second brain, novel interpretations concerning its function were hypothesized. This led to the writing of books and articles to divulge the concept that we have an extension of our brain inside our gut that sometimes works in a manner that was not envisaged before. For example, *Scientific American* in 2010 published an article entitled "Think Twice: How the Gut's "Second Brain" Influences Mood and

Well-Being" describing "The emerging and surprising view of how the enteric nervous system in our bellies goes far beyond just processing the food we eat". On the other side of the Atlantic, the BBC news in 2012 published an article by Michael Mosley, entitled "The second brain in our stomachs", which states that, "… new research is revealing the surprising ways in which our guts exert control over our mood and appetite".

Apart from the number of articles and books published on the subject, researchers in the fields of psychiatry, neurology and development look seriously into the function of the second brain to elucidate the pathogenesis of diseases that, until recently, were supposed to be diseases of the brain inside our heads. For example, a scientific article published in 2010 by researchers in psychiatry in the authoritative journal "Brain Behavior and Immunity"[2] and aptly entitled "Mood and gut feelings", concludes stating that "It may be that we need to change the focus from the brain and look at the role of the gut in what have traditionally been thought of as brain-based disorders".

According to another review on the subject:

> "The concept that the gut and the brain are closely connected, and that this interaction plays an important part not only in gastrointestinal function but also in certain feeling states and in intuitive decision making, is deeply rooted in our language. Recent neurobiological insights into this gut-brain crosstalk have revealed a complex, bidirectional communication system that not

---

2. 2010 Jan; 24(1):9-16

only ensures the proper maintenance of gastrointestinal homeostasis and digestion but is likely to have multiple effects on affect, motivation and higher cognitive functions, including intuitive decision making. Moreover, disturbances of this system have been implicated in a wide range of disorders, including functional and inflammatory gastrointestinal disorders, obesity and eating disorders."[3]

Therefore, we may summarize that our brain is partly inside our skull and partly outside our heads, notably in the walls of the GI tract, and all the parts of our brain cooperate in our processes of thoughts. But this is only the tip of the iceberg. In fact, both the brain inside our head and that in the GI tract are made of human neurons; that is, they are made of cells that pertain to the human part of our body and therefore can be aptly designated our "human brains". The instructions for the functioning of those human neurons are encoded in our human DNA, which contains approximately 22,000 genes, many of which regulate the behavior of those neurons.

Those 22,000 human genes are only one 360th of the genes that are within our (not-so-) human body. In fact, altogether, the mass of commensal or symbiotic microbes in our body, the microbiota, according to the NIH Microbiome Project, contains more than 360 times the total genetic material contained in all the cells in the human body, and therefore we are forced to acknowledge the existence of a third brain that this time is not only an extension or another anatomical part of the brain inside our head, but something completely

---

3. *Nat Rev Neurosci.* 2011 Jul 13; 12(8):453-66

different. It is a non-human brain that plays a role as important as the human brain in determining who we are and why we are doing what we are doing.

3

The Discovery of The Third Brain: "The Eureka Moment"

The mission of "The New Health Conversation" is to introduce you to what is available. We feel it is our job to peel back the layers and expose you to ideas, theories, new technologies and the overall evolution of how we view the human body. In this third book in "The New Health Conversation™" series, we are exploring one of the most incredible discoveries in history. This discovery will make you aware that it is only impossible until it is possible.

We must warn you that, to many, this will seem like science fiction. We assure you it is not. The scientific evidence is so overwhelming that everything we thought we knew about health, wellness, and what it means to be human will never be the same again. As you learned in the previous chapter, the discovery of the second brain has already had wide-ranging positive effects on wellness. In particular, the treatment of psychological conditions by psychiatrists has shifted from the brain in our heads to the gut itself.

The discovery of the second brain allowed doctors to interact with the gut to help so many plagued with mental illnesses. The realization that the microbiome is a third brain opened up a new dialogue for doctors to interact with this amazing organ to further enhance our wellness potential and our quality of life.

This third brain, as termed by Dr. Ruggiero, has everything to do with who we are, what we are, and what is possible for mankind. Dr. Ruggiero will present here the hard scientific evidence for the existence of the third brain.

THE THIRD BRAIN IN LAYMAN'S TERMS

When Dr. Ruggiero first introduced this concept, we were mystified, to say the least. It seemed like science fiction. Due to the complexity of the subject matter, we believe it is important to first give you a layman's version of the third brain as we understand it.

In the simplest terms, the microbiome is comprised of trillions of bacteria, viruses, fungi, yeasts, parasites and unknown microbes. Nearly 70% of the microbiome is contained and directly hot-wired, if you will, to the neurons that make up the second brain (the lining of the GI Tract). The other 30% of the microbiome is disbursed throughout the body in sinus cavities, blood, skin, and tear ducts.

The microbiome is created at birth when a baby comes into the world, at which point it is for the most part sterile. In natural childbirth, the baby picks up bacteria, viruses, fungi and yeast as it passes through the birth canal. Then, the mother begins to breastfeed the baby, first with colostrum (the clear liquid before breast milk rich in immunogenic proteins and healthy glycosaminoglycans) and then with the introduction of breast milk.

As Dr. Ruggiero and his colleagues discovered, a very compli-cated process occurs as the colostrum and mother's breast milk begin a fermentation process, while at the same time interacting with the fungi, yeast and bacteria, parasites, and unknown microbes that the baby picks up as it passes through the birth canal. In particular, a group of approximately 40 bacteria play a crucial and critical role in this process to create the microbiome. The formation of the intact microbiome takes two to three years.

Once fully formed, the microbiome becomes, in essence, the operating system for the human body. It is like a computer that is brand new with the best memory, hard drive and processors. This computer, however, is completely useless and will not function unless or until the Windows™-like operating system is installed. Once this operating system is completely installed and fully intact, the body can perform as intended. The ideal outcome—a fully physically, socially and emotionally intact human.

This is exactly the same concept as the microbiome. It is only when the microbiome is completely installed over a period of time that the human body has the ability to reach its maximum human potential. Many of you might be asking: What if the mother had a caesarian birth, or if the child is not breastfed?

Researchers have shown that cesarean born babies have higher incidences of allergies and behavioral issues later in life. The rea-son they believe this is because the baby has less exposure to the microbes, bacteria, yeast and fungi at birth than a baby born through a vaginal delivery. Although the ideal situation is for a mother to breast feed so that the colostrum and breast milk can ferment and form the microbiome, a child will be able to develop a microbiome through formula (that simulates breast milk) and from the microbes from our environment.

THE THIRD BRAIN IN MARCO'S WORDS

Dr. Marco Ruggiero: "In 2009, I received a grant from the Italian Ministry University to study the development of the brain from primates to humans. It was a research project of national interest, and it involved four other Universities in Italy along with a number of researchers (Protocol 2009LFSNAN). The goal of this project was to identify the genetic information that was responsible for the differences between apes and humans. What is it that makes the human brain and the human mind so different and so peculiar? In those days, it was thought that the main difference was due to the size of the brain and therefore in the number of connections that could be established between neurons. It was believed that the more connections, the more complex the workings of the brain and the mind. In simpler words, apes have smaller brains; therefore, they can process less information, and because of this, they cannot speak."

DR. RUGGIERO DISCOVERS RESEARCH OF A MAN MISSING 90% OF HIS FIRST BRAIN LIVES A PERFECTLY NORMAL LIFE

However, I knew that this was only part of the story and probably not the most important part. In fact, it had been demonstrated several years earlier that humans can live without 90% of the brain and can still perform all the complex tasks that humans are supposed to, including being a civil servant in the tax office in Marseille, France.

This incredible case was published in the very prestigious medical journal "The Lancet."[4]

This gentleman was married, had two children and lived a perfectly normal life. Every day he would drive in the chaotic traffic of Marseille to go to work. It was quite an accidental discovery that about 90% of his brain was missing and, essentially, his skull was filled with liquid. This liquid is normally in minute quantities in the brain ventricles. And this is not the only case of a person living a normal life without having a brain inside the head. Even though these observations went completely unnoticed in the medical/scientific community, in 1992, Berker (*et al.*) had observed that in twins, the one of the two with drastically reduced cerebral cortex size showed above-average intelligence.[5]

In other words, it appears that not only is the brain in our heads not the end all be all (please notice, there is no other organ that can be 90% absent and still not cause any limitation or disease), but that the less brain tissue we have, the more intelligent we may be. I agree that these statements may appear "brainless" or better yet downright crazy, but these are the hard facts of science.

4. Feuillet L, Dufour H, Pelletier J. Lancet. 2007 Jul 21; 370(9583):262. "A Man with 90% of his First Brain Missing"

5. Dev Med Child Neurol. 1992 Jul;34(7):623-32. Reciprocal neurological developments of twins discordant for hydrocephalus. Berker E, Goldstein G, Lorber J, Priestley B, Smith A

GENETIC INFORMATION IS THE KEY TO BRAIN FUNCTION

Now, knowing the differences in the size and histological structure of the brain between apes and humans might not have been so relevant at the time. Since we now understood there can be humans without 90% of their brain who still are perfectly functioning humans, I focused my attention and the attention of my very bright collaborators toward the concept of genetic information. We looked at genetic information to determine if it was actually responsible for the working of the brain and, consequently, of the mind. Here, we made some interesting observations by using sophisticated methods of computational analysis that allowed us to compare the genetic information in apes and humans.

The starting point was the observation that the acquisition of articulated language as a system of communication, which was strictly and exclusively human, was certainly a turning point in human evolution. Paleoanthropologists can be certain of only two factors related directly and indirectly to articulated language. The first is that it is evident that articulated language differentiates *Homo sapiens* from all other living beings. Only humans are capable of using a complex verbal language both as a means of communication and as an instrument for introspective reflection. The second is that the brain of *Homo sapiens* is about three times larger than that of our closest relatives, in evolutionary terms, *i.e.*, the African ape. On the basis of the observation that humans can live with almost no brain and still retain the ability to speak, we are now certain there can be little relationship between these two observations.

Previously, a group of researchers at the U.S. National Institutes on Deafness and Other Communication Disorders identified three mutations in the gene designated GNPTG, which encodes the gamma subunit of the GNPT protein, in stuttering subjects of Asian and European descent but not in control subjects. Furthermore, they identified three mutations in another gene, the NAGPA gene, which encodes the so-called "uncovering enzyme", in other stuttering subjects but not in control subjects.

Therefore, the purpose of our research was to compare the sequences of the genes NAGPA, GNPTAB and GNPTG in species where the nucleotide sequences of the entire genome, relevant to human evolution, are known as: *Homo sapiens, Pan Troglodytes, Pongo spp, Macaca mulatta, Mus musculus, Equus caballus, Gallus domesticus, Taeniopygia guttata* and *Danio rerio.*

After having compared the nucleotide and amino-acid sequences, we had finally identified, for all the studied genes, the amino-acid substitutions that were most important from a functional point of view. However, evolutionary analysis on the genes evidenced no sign of positive selection. This latter observation was quite puzzling, since it appeared that there was no evolutionary advantage in learning to speak, something that goes completely against common sense.

Therefore, we were facing not one, but two conundrums: humans can live intelligent lives without brains, and the genes coding for speech were not under evolutionary selection.

THE EUREKA MOMENT

I remember that it was a very ordinary morning, during the most ordinary of our daily meetings that we had in the library of the Department of Biochemical Sciences at the University of Firenze, when a completely crazy idea came to light in my mind. Professor Brunetto Chiarelli, a brilliant anthropologist who had recently retired, was talking about the different anatomical areas of the human brain, and he was focusing his talk on the so-called, "reptilian brain." This part of the brain is part of the triune brain that is a model of the evolution of the vertebrate forebrain and behavior as the American physician and neuroscientist, Paul D. MacLean, originally proposed it. MacLean formulated his model in the 1960s and published it at length in his 1990 book, "The Triune Brain in Evolution". The triune brain consists of the reptilian complex, the paleo mammalian complex (limbic system), and the neo-mammalian complex (neocortex), viewed as structures sequentially added to the forebrain over the course of evolution. However, it has to be said that the majority of comparative neuroscientists no longer accept this hypothesis in the post-2000 era.

COULD THE BRAIN IN OUR HEAD BE NONHUMAN?

While I was thinking of the reptilian brain with, I must say, little attention, I wondered whether, by any chance, our brain was actually non-human. My reasoning in that lazy and rather boring meeting was: If the brain is based on genetic information, as it is, and if the majority of the genetic information in our body is non-human (*i.e.* it's in the microbiome), then the logical corollary should be that the majority of our brain should be in the information contained in the microbiome and, hence, not human.

I immediately realized the revolutionary potential of this intuition! I stopped listening to Professor Chiarelli and immediately began to search for contradictions in such a revolutionary hypothesis. As of today, I have not been able to find one. Therefore, since the term "the second brain" had already been coined, I thought that this one could have been aptly named "the third brain".

The concept of the third brain, like many other concepts in biology and medicine, has not been the invention or the discovery of a single author. It rather emerged from a combination of observations that are ultimately changing the perspective of our position as humans in the biological universe.

In fact, the discovery and the characterization of the human microbiome led to a revolution in our way of interpreting our role in the universe that is paralleled only by the two major scientific and cultural revolutions of the past centuries. The first of these revolutions occurred when Copernicus, Galileo and Kepler downgraded the position of our earth from the center of the universe to a rather astronomically irrelevant position in the physical universe. The second occurred when Darwin demonstrated that humans were not a sort of privileged species, but rather the product of an ongoing process of biological evolution that applies to all living beings on this earth since the appearance of the first living cell. And the third revolution that can be interpreted as a blow to our self-declared human superiority in the biological world is occurring right now: the discovery that many, if not all of our supposedly superior neuropsychological intelligence is in reality influenced or straightforwardly manipulated by a non-human part of our body, the microbiome.

It's interesting to note that the concept of the microbiome emerged shortly after the characterization of the human genome and, as a matter of fact, the suffix "ome" derives from the information that we gathered from studying the human genome. The current definition of the human genome, as we can find it in Wikipedia, is "The human genome is the complete set of genetic information for humans (*Homo sapiens sapiens*). This information is encoded as DNA sequences within the 23 chromosome in cell nuclei and in a small DNA molecule found within individual mitochondria". According to this definition, the genetic information for humans is encoded in about 22,000 genes that are responsible for the synthesis and functions of all our proteins and hence all of our cells and ultimately all of our organs, including the brain.

WHAT IS GENETIC INFORMATION AND WHY IS IT SO IMPORTANT?

Genetic information is the basis of all living forms in this planet, and it is based on the concept of "gene". According to some interpretations, the word gene is derived from the Greek word *genesis,* meaning birth, or *genos,* meaning "origin"; however, according to other interpretations, the word gene derives from the Latin "gens", and it indicates family, hence familiarity or heredity. As a matter of fact, since the fifties, it was demonstrated that a gene is the molecular unit of heredity of a living organism. Living beings depend on genes, i.e. those stretches of DNA that hold the information to build and maintain an organism's cells and pass genetic traits to offspring.

All organisms have genes corresponding to various biological traits, some of which are instantly visible, such as eye color or number of limbs, and some of which are not, such as blood type, increased risk for specific diseases, or the thousands of basic biochemical processes that comprise life.

Note that the keywords in this definition are what is called *genetic information*. In fact, in modern days, the concept of genetic information has transcended the boundaries of biological sciences, and it has been adopted and elaborated by philosophers to describe life itself. The most comprehensive definition of life nowadays is that of "genetic information that replicates itself and is transmitted in time". Therefore, we may safely conclude that human life could be defined as the information contained in our genome (22,000 human genes). In other words, our life was interpreted as the genetic information contained in our human DNA.

ONLY LESS THAN ONE PERCENT OF OUR GENES ARE HUMAN

All this might have satisfied our understanding of human life until the discovery and characterization of the human genome. Thus, it was demonstrated in The Microbiome Project (National Institute of Health Research) that inside our body there are about 8,000,000 genes, out of which only 22,000 are those of the human genome. In other words, bona fide human genes account only for less than 1% of the whole genetic information that we carry with us. The other more than 99% of the genetic information pertains to the microbes forming our microbiome. Therefore, if we share the consensus that "ife" is genetic information, then we have to deduce that our genetic information, *i.e.* our life itself, is less than 1% human.

REDEFINING MIND AND FREE WILL

This sort of downgrading bears even worse consequences for our human ego, even more so than simply being put in a corner of the galaxy as Copernicus did. In fact, the consequences of this realization reach far beyond the realm of probiotics and gut flora and force us to redefine even the concepts of mind and free will. But let's try to follow some order and to put this information in perspective.

Up until now, it was thought that the information for the function of our cells and organs, including the neurons and the brain was encoded in our DNA by those 22,000 genes that constitute our genome. Since it had been demonstrated scientifically that the neurons in our brains formed connections that exchanged electrochemical information through the synapses, it was thought that the working of our mind was based on those neuronal-interconnections and the exchange of electrochemical signals.[6]

The organization of the neuronal interconnections and, hence, the cellular and molecular bases for the working of our mind is like plastic and adapts to the different situations that lead to learning and memorizing concepts that are functional for our survival and well-being. All these features are encoded in our human DNA and, therefore, pertain to our human brains.

---

6. Front Hum Neurosci. 2014 Oct 13;8:815. doi: 10.3389/fnhum.2014.00815. eCollection 2014. Meeting the brain on its own terms. Haueis P

WHAT IS INFORMATION? UNDERSTANDING OUR NON-HUMAN BRAIN

Here, we have to enter in depth into the definition of "information" if we wish to understand why our non-human third brain, an organ completely missed for millennia, is so important in all our neurological and psychological processes. In fact, there are two systems of information that are superimposed and that have to be coherent, (isomorphic) as in formal logics following the principles enunciated by the Austrian-British philosopher Ludwig Josef Johann Wittgenstein.

In his 75-page *Tractatus Logico-Philosophicus* of 1921, Wittgenstein essentially states that the world (*i.e.* the objective reality), the mind that perceives and interprets the world, and the language that is used by the mind to describe the world, contain the same information. Therefore, if one wishes to study the world, he or she only has to study the language that describes such a world, since the information contained in the world, in the mind and in the language, has the same meaning even though the nature of the information in itself may be different.

WHAT IS DNA?

DNA, or deoxyribonucleic acid, is the hereditary material in humans and almost all other organisms. Nearly every cell in a person's body has the same DNA. Most DNA is located in the cell nucleus (where it is called nuclear DNA), but a small amount of DNA can also be found in the mitochondria (where it is called mitochondrial DNA or mt DNA).

The information in DNA is stored as a code made up of four chemical bases: adenine (A), guanine (G), cytosine (C), and thymine (T). Human DNA consists of about three billion bases, and more than 99% of those bases are the same in all people. The order, or sequence, of these bases determines the information available for building and maintaining an organism, similar to the way in which letters of the alphabet appear in a certain order to form words and sentences.

DNA bases pair up with each other, A with T and C with G, to form units called base pairs. Each base is also attached to a sugar molecule and a phosphate molecule. Together, a base, sugar, and phosphate are called a nucleotide. Nucleotides are arranged in two long strands that form a spiral called a double helix. The structure of the double helix is somewhat like a ladder, with the base pairs forming the ladder's rungs and the sugar and phosphate molecules forming the vertical sidepieces of the ladder.

An important property of DNA is that it can replicate (make copies of itself). Each strand of DNA in the double helix can serve as a pattern for duplicating the sequence of bases. This is critical when cells divide, because each new cell needs to have an exact copy of the DNA present in the old cell.

DNA is a double helix formed by base pairs attached to a sugar-phosphate backbone.

FOR MORE INFORMATION ABOUT DNA:

The National Human Genome Research Institute fact sheet Deoxyribonucleic Acid (DNA) provides an introduction to this molecule:

> This concept is at the basis of modern molecular biology
> even though most molecular biologists have never heard
> of Wittgenstein. In fact, the information in the sequence
> of bases in DNA, RNA and in the sequence of amino-acids
> in proteins is essentially the same, isomorphic, even
> though the chemical nature of DNA, RNA and proteins is
> different.

Therefore, in perfect accordance with Wittgenstein, if one wishes to study the information contained in a gene, (in DNA that, in Wittgenstein's view, could be the world), he could study the protein (the language), which is exactly what most molecular biologists do. And it is not coincidence, or if it is a coincidence, it is of the type described by Jung, that these biochemical processes are called "transcription" and "translation", indicating the flow of isomorphic information from DNA to RNA and from RNA to proteins, respectively.

In our quest to understand the third brain, remember that one system of information is the genetic information contained in our DNA. In other words, this is the basic information of life that is shared by all living beings on this earth. Here, there is a sequence of bases in the DNA that codes for (different) bases in the RNA that are then translated in sequences of amino-acids that form proteins, which in turn form cells.

This is an example of DNA sequencing: A small nucleotide sequence is, for example, (CGGGTACGAAT). Its complementary sequence would be (GCCCATGCTTA).

DNA INFORMATION DETERMINES THE SHAPE AND FUNCTION OF OUR CELLS

The shape and the function of a cell and, therefore, of an organism, are due to this information contained in the DNA, in our case, in our human DNA. The information remains the same even though it is translated into different molecules (bases and amino-acids), exactly as it happens when a language is translated into another. The sequence of the letters in the words is different, but the meaning remains the same. This is what happens to our biological information, which is contained in our DNA and, through a long and complex series of passages, is translated into a living being. It is important to remember that the information may change shape, but its meaning has to remain the same, and this is the very concept of isomorphism.

NEURONAL INTERCONNECTIONS SECOND SYSTEM OF INFORMATION IN OUR HUMAN BRAINS

We have another system of information that is due to the neuronal interconnections in our human brains. Here, we have cells that exchange electrochemical signals just as happens in computer chips. But, unlike computer chips that are "fixed", these neuronal interconnections are flexible and plastic, because they have to adapt to the changing environment. This type of information underlies our processes of learning, memory, decision-making, mood control and all the neuropsychological function that we know.

HOW IS INFORMATION IN OUR DNA RELATED TO INFORMATION IN OUR HUMAN BRAINS?

The question is: how is the system of information contained in the DNA related to the system of information due to the neuronal interconnections in our brains? Are the two systems isomorphic? Or, in other words, does our DNA determine our thoughts? Until recently, this was the assumption. Therefore, I could have said that I was intelligent or not, able to play piano or not, shy or exuberant, because of my genes contained in my DNA. And this, of course, took into account the influence of the environment, because the way we react to the environment is due to the information contained in our DNA, which makes us more or less able to adapt to specific changes. This is the classical Darwinian theory of evolution with the survival of the fittest, though not certainly of the strongest. The ability to adapt, contained in our genes, is the key to survival. And this adaptability obviously encompasses the ability to adapt our neuronal interconnection so as to better cope with an environment that is constantly changing.

TWO SYSTEMS OF INFORMATION DNA AND OUR BRAINS

If we now try to understand these concepts at the light of Wittgenstein's theory, we have two systems of information, the one in our DNA and the one in our brains, that are isomorphic, coherent and superimposable; therefore, if we understand one of the two systems, we automatically and by definition also understand the other one. And since it is much easier to study DNA rather than the functioning of our human brains, much attention has been devoted to the study of the genes in DNA. In summary: the information contained in the DNA determines our ability to process the information in our heads, and the two systems of information are isomorphic and coherent, to the joy of the philosophers.

Some tiny molecules and some tiny non-human cells, however, just like the proverbial grain of dust in the machinery, clog the entire philosophical system and force us to redefine the whole concept of brain and mind and to move away from Wittgenstein's interpretation and enter into the realm of Kurt Goedel's mathematical philosophy.

Kurt Friedrich Goedel was an Austrian logician, mathematician, and philosopher who moved to Princeton at the beginning of World War II. He is considered, along with Aristotle and Gottlob Frege, one of the most significant logicians in the history of mankind. He made an immense impact upon scientific and philosophical thinking in the 20th century by publishing his two incompleteness theorems in 1931, when he was 25 years old.

The technique that he developed to demonstrate his theorems, known as Goedel's numbering, is at the basis of the functioning of modern computers, including this one on which I am writing. The incompleteness theorems are among the most complex and fascinating mathematical topics, and there is no hope to understand them in their most profound meaning without a high grade of competence in mathematics and logics.

Just to give an example, the first theorem states that for any self-consistent recursive axiomatic system powerful enough to describe the arithmetic of the natural numbers, there are true propositions about the naturals that cannot be proved from the axioms. In layman's terms, this theorem demonstrates that every system of information, including those described above, is incomplete by definition, and there are statements that the system cannot designate as true or false.

GOEDEL'S THEOREMS AND THEIR RELATIONSHIP TO THE THIRD BRAIN

How do Goedel's theorems apply to our understanding of the third brain? What is the nature of the tiny particle of dust that demonstrates that the systems are incomplete? These figurative particles of dust are small molecules, called neurotransmitters, that are responsible for the signaling between neurons and determine all of our neuropsychological functions.

ELECTRO CHEMICAL SIGNALS

When we describe the transmission of signals through our neuronal network, we use the term "electrochemical"; this means that the neurons produce and release small molecules (hence the term "chemical") called neurotransmitters that induce an electrical signal, called depolarization, of the receiving cell membrane. The electrical signal is always of the same nature in all cells, and it can be only positive or negative (hyper- or depolarization). The chemical signal, however, i.e. the chemical nature of the neurotransmitter, is highly variable, and there are many neurotransmitters with different chemical structures. Dopamine, serotonin, noradrenaline, acetylcholine, and GABA are just a few examples of neurotransmitters with very distinguished chemical structures.

NEUROTRANSMITTERS ARE RESPONSIBLE FOR FUNCTIONING OF OUR FIRST BRAIN

Neurotransmitters are produced by the neurons and the information to produce one or another neurotransmitter. Each one has very different effects on the receiving cell behavior, which is encoded in the cell's DNA, in our case in the human DNA that "tells" the human neuron which neurotransmitters produce, and when, for how long and how much they do. Up until now, everything seems simple and in perfect accordance with Wittgenstein's theory of systems isomorphism. The information encoded in the DNA is responsible for the production of a neurotransmitter, and this neurotransmitter is responsible for the functioning of our human brains.

The fundamental role of the neurotransmitters in all our neuro-psychological function is widely acknowledged by pharmacology (prescription drugs), that by manipulating the production of neurotransmitters, we can influence the working of our brains. For example, serotonin is responsible for the regulation of pleasure, concentration, mood, appetite, and sleep, and it is involved in our cognitive functions, including memory and learning. When the serotonin signal is not working properly, ADD, ADHD, depression, obsessive-compulsive disorder and anxiety ensue. Therefore, modulation of serotonin at synapses is one of the major actions of several classes of pharmacological antidepressants. Conversely, when the serotonin signal works properly, there is a feeling of happiness and wellbeing. And, according to the authoritative *Journal of Psychiatry and Neurosciences*, "happiness and well-being are important, both as factors protecting against mental and physical disorders and in their own right. Conversely, negative moods are associated with negative outcomes. For example, the negative mood hostility is a risk factor for many disorders."[7]

Simplifying to the extreme, we may say that our genes are responsible for the serotonin signaling that makes us happy or depressed, in a state of well-being or of anxiety, and these mental states then influence our overall health. This reasoning will apply to all neurotransmitters that regulate all our cerebral functions. In Wittgenstein's type of systems, the information in our DNA is isomorphic (identical or similar) to the functioning of our brains, and therefore, the information in our DNA *is* our brains.

NON-HUMAN GENETIC INFORMATION IS THE BASIS FOR THE THIRD BRAIN

This deterministic, and rather frightening, vision could be true if in our body there was only the information encoded in our human DNA, that is the information in the approximately 22,000 human genes. But we already know that in our bodies, there are 8,000,000 other, non-human genes that pertain to the microbes constituting the microbiome. Since the genetic information in DNA is always the same in all living beings, we can now understand how this enormous, non-human genetic information that is with us since the moment we are born accounts for a third brain.

The third brain, in essence, is the DNA information of the more than 8,000,000 non-human genes in our body. That is what makes it a third brain, as the microbiome has vast stores of DNA information that play a vital role in human beings.

---

7. J Psychiatry Neurosci. 2007 Nov; 32(6): 394–399

It should now be clear why the massive array of fungi, bacteria, viruses and yeast's 8,000,000 genes has such an overwhelming influence on our quality of life potential. Keep in mind that for more than (this should not be here) 3,000 years of study of human anatomy, this microbiome (the third brain) went undetected.

DEFINING THE THIRD BRAIN

We now have all the elements to define the third brain. In a perfectly coherent isomorphism that would delight both Wittgenstein and Goedel, the third brain is the array of microbes that constitute the microbiome, which contains the genetic information constituted by 8,000,000 genes.

At this point, one may wonder how these non-human genes exchange their information with the human genes and where the point of contact is at which these two systems of information, the human and the non-human, communicate with each other.

POINT OF CONTACT FOR HUMAN AND NON-HUMAN GENES

The point of contact is constituted by the neurotransmitters; in fact, microbes of the microbiome have encoded in their DNA the information to produce and release the very same neurotransmitters that are responsible for our mental states. For example, they – the microbes – may produce the serotonin that makes us happy and in a state of wellbeing and, most intriguingly, our happiness and wellbeing is very positive for the microbes themselves and increases their probability of survival.

DECISION MAKING IS DONE IN THE THIRD BRAIN

It may sound strange, but our behavior, our mental states, our feelings are not born inside our heads, but rather inside our guts, where the majority of microbes reside. And it is quite possible that we have little free will, with most of our decision-making capabilities attributed to the information contained in the third brain. The third brain, therefore, becomes the proposition that cannot be proven in Goedel's theorem.

Neuroscientists are becoming accustomed to the concept that this other system of information actually manipulates our entire behavior, and they are using this verb, "manipulate", in their austere scientific publications.

For example, in his recently published article entitled "Microbes on the edge of Occam's razor" Dr. Starokadomskyy of the Department of Internal Medicine, UT Southwestern Medical Center in Dallas, writes:

> "Our body harbors hundreds of microbial species and contains many more bacteria than human cells. These microbes are not passive riders but rather a vital component of the organism. The human microbiota affects our health in multiple ways, both positively and negatively. One of the new attractive directions in microbiome biology is the "microbiome-brain axis".

Several groups of researchers have described the ability of the gut microbiota to communicate with the brain and thus modulate human behavior."[8]

---

8. *Biol Direct.* 2014 Nov 30;10(1):25

Other researchers define the relationship between microbes and the human brains as a paradigm shift in neuroscience[9] and write:

> "The discovery of the size and complexity of the human microbiome has resulted in an ongoing reevaluation of many concepts of health and disease, including diseases affecting the central nervous system. A growing body of preclinical literature has demonstrated bidirectional signaling between the brain and the gut microbiome, involving multiple neurocrine and endocrine signaling mechanisms... experimental changes to the gut microbiome can affect emotional behavior and related brain systems. These findings have resulted in speculation that alterations in the gut microbiome may play a pathophysiological role in human brain diseases, including autism spectrum disorder, anxiety, depression, and chronic pain."

It is important to notice that this article, published in November 2014, clearly states that changing the gut microbiome may result in changes in emotional behavior and related brain systems. And this is the scientific basis for the development of types of food that, in actuality, are transplants of genetic information or transplants of the third brain.

Another article published at about the same time, in October 2014, uses the phrase "to manipulate" and states that our eating behavior is manipulated by the microbiome to make us eat what goes

9. J Neurosci. 2014 Nov 12; 34(46):15490-6. Gut microbes and the brain: paradigm shift in neuroscience. Mayer EA, Knight R, Mazmanian SK, Cryan JF, Tillisch K

to their advantage (and not necessarily ours). The title of the article leaves no room for doubts: "Is eating behavior manipulated by the gastrointestinal microbiota? "Evolutionary pressures and potential mechanisms."[10] In this article, Alcock et al. unequivocally state that microbes manipulate our eating patterns.

> "Microbes in the gastrointestinal tract are under selective pressure to manipulate host eating behavior to increase their fitness, sometimes at the expense of host fitness. Microbes may do this through two potential strategies: i.e. generating cravings for foods that they specialize on or foods that suppress their competitors, or (ii) inducing dysphoria until we eat foods that enhance their fitness."

This means that it is not us who decide what we like to eat, but rather the microbes that decide for us what to eat, and they do this to enhance their fitness, not necessarily ours. Thus, we may have already lost a great deal of our supposed free will; in fact, the eating behavior is the most fundamental of all behaviors, since it is the behavior designed by evolution to keep us alive. It has been said before that food matters. Now that statement needs to be expanded to make sure that when we are eating, we are supplying the best food possible for our three brains.

If our microbiome is not fed properly, the human part of us will not be at its highest quality of life, even if we eat organic and exercise regularly. It has now become more apparent than ever that what we

10. Bioessays. 2014 Oct; 36(10):940-9

put in our mouths affects a universe that we recently had no idea even existed.

MICROBES HAVE EMOTIONS

If you thought that microbes have no emotions, then the title of this article, published in the austere *Neurogastroenterology and Motility Journal*[11] may surprise you: "Melancholic microbes: a link between gut microbiota and depression?". In this article, the Authors clearly write:

> "There is a growing awareness of the potential for microbiota to influence gut-brain communication in health and disease. A variety of strategies have been used to study the impact of the microbiota on brain function and these include antibiotic use, probiotic treatments, fecal microbiota transplantation, gastrointestinal infection studies, and germ-free studies. All of these approaches provide evidence to support the view that the microbiota can influence brain chemistry and consequently behavior. ... This has direct implications for the development of psychobiotic-based therapeutic strategies for psychiatric disorders."

This last sentence bears an enormous implication not only for psychiatric disorders, but also for the ultimate functioning of our three brains. If we use Goedel's logics, we shall be able to regain our precious free will. Before we can do this, we still have to learn how

---

11. 2013 Sep; 25(9):713-9

the third brain manipulates us and what the implications of this for health and disease are.

Together with Authors Louis and Flint, we have to learn "How our gut microbes influence our behavior[12] and realize that:

> "... Gut bacteria help to maintain a healthy intestine by providing nutrients and guarding against pathogens. Recent evidence, however, suggests that their actions reach beyond the gut, as they appear to influence various aspects of host physiology, ranging from the regulation of food intake to behavior and mood. Bacteria and their metabolites can interact with the host via routes involving the immune, nervous and endocrine system."

We also have to consider that the third brain corruption is evident in a variety of different conditions. The connection between the microbial third brain and the development of the human brain is clearly evident in the neurodevelopmental disorder known as Autism.

At the beginning of 2015, Toh and Allen-Vercoe of the Department of Molecular and Cellular Biology of University of Guelph in Canada published an article entitled: "The human gut microbiota with reference to autism spectrum disorder: considering the whole as more than a sum of its parts", where they wrote that, basically, the third brain is now recognized as a critical component of the highest quality of life.

---

12. J Neuroendocrinology. 2013 May; 25(5):517-8

"The human gut microbiota is a complex microbial
ecosystem that contributes an important component
towards the health of its host. This highly complex
ecosystem has been underestimated in its importance
until recently, when a realization of the enormous scope
of gut microbiota function has been (and continues to be)
revealed. One of the more striking of these discoveries
is the finding that the gut microbiota and the brain are
connected, and thus there is potential for the microbiota
in the gut to influence behavior and mental health. In
this short review, we outline the link between brain
and gut microbiota and urge the reader to consider
the gut microbiota as an ecosystem 'organ' rather than
just as a collection of microbes filling a niche, using
the hypothesized role of the gut microbiota in autism
spectrum disorder to illustrate the concept."[13]

The microbiome manipulates all aspects of behavior, health,
and disease.

All this novel scientific information published in prestigious
peer-reviewed journals that are indexed in the PubMed, the database of the National Library of Medicine of the National Institutes of
Health of the USA, can be summarized as follows: the genetic information in the microbiome, those 8,000,000 non-human genes in our
bodies, manipulates all the aspects of our behavior and is responsible
for our states of health and disease, and our potential quality of life.

---

13. Microb Ecol Health Dis. 2015 Jan 28; 26:26309.

99% OF OUR INFORMATION IS NON-HUMAN (MICROBIAL)

Stated as such, this may not seem to be very encouraging news. There is something else to be considered if we keep on following this logic: if the information in DNA is the key to describing life itself and the functioning of our brains (both human and nonhuman), and if we, as human beings, are a symbiosis of human and non-human genes, then it only seems logical that 99% of our information is microbial (8,000,000 microbial genes versus 22,000 human genes). Our human information is definitely in the minority as far as sheer numbers are concerned, but it may not be so unimportant.

Can we interact with this microbial world? What if we could manipulate the microbes that manipulate us? We would acquire a much higher degree of free will, much higher than before when we were led to believe, erroneously, that all the processes of decision-making occurred in our human brains.

This concept is stated, in embryonic form, in the sentence published in the *Neurogastroenterology and Motility Journal* hypothesizing the "development of psychobiotic-based therapeutic strategies for psychiatric disorders". In essence, this sentence states that if we understand how the microbiome influences our behavior in health and disease, we may decide to change the microbiome and, therefore, to introduce into ourselves those microbes that contain the information that is instrumental to our health, happiness and well-being. "Psychobiotic" here indicates microbes that manipulate our behavior. It implies that we may decide which are the microbes that are good for us and which are bad.

DISCOVERY OF FOOD FOR THE THIRD BRAIN

With the evidence building that we can actually influence the third brain, we started to look at the fuels that could sustain and strengthen the microbiome. This is what led to the search for the right type of nourishment for the microbiome. We were looking for much more than food—we were looking for fuel that could manipulate the genetic information in the third brain itself. After many different recipes and formulations, we discovered the food for the microbiome and why the third brain must consume it. Our theories and discoveries suggest that the third brain must have proper nourishment in order to maximize our quality of life. Nourishment must be provided not just for our bellies, but for our 22,000 human genes and 8,000,000 non-human genes as well.

FOOD IS INFORMATION

Food, in addition to providing us with calories and nutrients, provides us with genetic information. Food's genetic make-up adds to existing genetic information that already exists in our body. Food is not sterile and contains an enormous array of microbes that bring information to our bodies. It is quite fascinating that some of these nutrients are beneficial for some microbes, while others are detrimental. Therefore, every time that we introduce some food into our body, we actually alter our microbiome. By doing so, we may also alter the messages sent to our brain.

At this point, we may decide that we want to introduce only those microbes that are beneficial for us, choosing foods that will keep us in good health. As evidenced above, the microbiome controls all the functions of all the organs, including, for example, the immune and endocrine systems. Therefore, we may decide to eat a food containing those microbes that contribute to the functioning of our immune system as well as all our system and apparatuses.

THE 35-YEAR SEARCH LEADING TO THE DISCOVERY OF THE SUPER MICROBES

Where do we find these microbes, and how can we make sure that they are in the food that we eat? This has been the object of Dr. Ruggiero's research for the past 35 years, since when he first started to study the role of food in health and disease. In a nutshell, we have to find out which are the microbial strains that constitute the healthy core human microbiome, the limited number of strains that we acquire when we are born and fed with the colostrum and milk from our mother's breast milk. Then, we have to reconstitute these strains in milk and colostrum exactly as they were when we were born *et voilà*! We have the healthy human core microbiome, the third brain, the directors of the immune and endocrine systems, in a cup that we can enjoy as a tasty dessert.

By introducing this food, we change our microbiome and we return to the primeval healthy state of our birth; our immune system will be ready to fight any challenge; our human brain will receive the information that is needed for its correct development and functioning, and so will all other organs and systems from the cardiovascular to the gastrointestinal. Does this sound like science fiction? Not really. For about 3,000 years, mankind has known that fermented milk products such as yogurts have beneficial effects on health and longevity, because fermented milk products reproduce what happens in our intestine when we were fed with our mothers' milk.

Once Dr. Ruggiero recognized the enormity of the microbiome, he concluded that this was, in fact, a true command center of our existence. Therefore, he deemed this entity the third brain. Upon this discovery, he and his team immediately began to figure out if there was a way to interact with this command center. If Dr. Ruggiero and his team could interact with the microbiome, it could be a new way to greatly enhance our ability to live healthier longer and improve life for so many people This is the amazing story of how Dr. Ruggiero realized that the microbiome was not only the third brain, but that it also plays a critical role in regulating and directing the functions of the immune system as well as of all the other organs of our body.

CORRUPTION OF THE THIRD BRAIN

We have established the concept of the third brain as the main command center for physical and emotional health. In a perfect world, things run smoothly. We have mental clarity, and our bodies run with the utmost of ease. But this world is not perfect. We do not live perfect lifestyles. We do not live in bubbles. If you have read the earlier books in "The New Health Conversation" Series, you have been educated about TDOS Syndrome. This is neither a disease nor a direct illness, but rather four *interconnected* components that are greatly involved in the disturbance of the third brain. The four components that prevent us from maximizing our wellness potential are toxicity, nutrient deficiency, overweightness, and stress.

TOXICITY

This refers to exposure of direct and indirect environmental substances that are deemed carcinogenic, poisonous or just not tolerated by the human body or microbiome. Such substances include artificial sweeteners, lead, heavy metals, herbicides, pesticides, etc. Even things that have been created to make us "healthier" can in fact wreak havoc on our bodies. Antibiotics, chemotherapy, and other medications affect our immune systems and gut health—causing a corrupt microbiome.

THE OVERUSE OF ANTIBIOTICS

We specifically positioned the use of antibiotics under toxicity due to overuse and its effect on the microbiome. The most damaging impact on the microbiome is the use or overuse of antibiotics. One of medicine's best and most-used discoveries has been antibiotics. Through these, we are able to rid the body of some harmful and even deadly bacterial infections. However, side effects from these strong antibiotics include stomach distress and imbalance of gut flora. Many doctors recommend utilizing a probiotic to combat this side effect.

Dr. Ruggiero and his colleagues have demonstrated that it is critical to not only recolonize the good gut flora, but to reconstitute the full microbiome, especially after finishing a round of antibiotic prescribed treatment. The microbiome is a major support and command center for our second brain and its immune system.

DEFICIENCY

This stands for nutrient deficiency: Due to over planting, lack of crop rotation, and the abundant overuse of herbicides and pesticides, our food no longer contains the nutrients and minerals it once did. Our bodies cannot perform optimally with inadequate nutrients and minerals. Food is no longer enough. We need to nourish our third brain.

OVERWEIGHT

Yes, our food is deficient in minerals and nutrients that allow for our bodies to be able to become fully nourished. This deficiency can lead to overeating. Without the nutrient balance in check and knowing that certain neurotransmitters are produced in our second brain (GI-tract), many overeat to fill a "happiness void". Our bodies look overfed, but are actually undernourished.

STRESS

As a society, we no longer have to hunt and gather. You can find food everywhere. Our bodies create cortisol for fight or flight situations. This is very much necessary for life. That being said, our hectic lifestyles cause us to produce way too much of this hormone. We need to manage this stress hormone in order to maintain our energy, maintain a healthy weight, and maintain a healthy psyche. As we have made the connection before, important neurotransmitters are created in the gut. An imbalance caused by stress can lead to gastric distress, depression, and a variety of other related symptoms.

So what happens when this command center gets corrupted? What happens when the supporting entities of the command center are compromised? What happens to our body? Well....

All of these contributing factors can lead to the corruption of the microbiome, as well as corruption in the cranial brain and the microbes in the GI tract.

Hundreds of years ago, we did not have the types of diseases we find today. The staggering number of people diagnosed with physical and psychological conditions and illnesses in the past few decades has been in epic proportion to what it was in the past. The numbers keep growing. It seems as if food allergies and intolerances are increasing annually. Not only is autism on the rise (it is estimated that approximately 1 in 68 children born are on the Autism Spectrum, up from 1 in 10,000 in 1990), but so are instances of children with developmental and social-emotional issues. Parents hop from therapist to therapist, filling prescription after prescription in efforts to treat the symptoms. We can put a bandage on a broken arm, or we can choose to repair the fracture by giving it what it truly needs to heal.

When the parts of a computer are weakened, the overall functioning of the system becomes sluggish; it does not perform optimally, and often times, shuts down completely. With the weakening of the command center, or hard drive, the system can be vulnerable to viruses and easily hacked.

But unlike a computer, where you can run to the Apple Store or Best Buy to get a new device or machine when it's broken, we need to be able to restore what is broken inside our bodies. To salvage the computer, it is likely that we will need to replace the hard drive, the command center, in order to restore the other parts and have a functioning machine again.

Our bodies work similarly. When we weaken our systems with the Standard American Diet and consuming substances that our bodies do not recognize or know how to process, knowingly or not, bad things can happen. Our bodies and minds are working on overdrive, with the family-work balance, eating on the run, the constant stress over money, and the pressure to perform.

The result? Like the computer, our bodies become sluggish: we catch viruses easily and are prone to damage in our own main control centers. Without intervention, TDOS Syndrome can only contribute to the demise of the microbiome.

"The New Health Conversation" brings to light what is now available. The solutions, if utilized correctly, will diminish the limiting impact TDOS Syndrome may have on our quality of life and our ability to maximize our wellness potential.

The good news is that Dr. Ruggiero and his team have been able to reconstitute the genetic information of the microbiome through their tireless research and the recreation of the fermentation process (including the 40-some strains of microbes) that occurs with natural birth and breastfeeding for all of us. This can help to fully optimize the microbiome, even in those who had cesarean births. In essence, the reconstitution of the genetic information of the microbiome is now possible on a continuing basis.

This major discovery has had great benefit already to maximize the quality of life for those who have been able to consume, for lack of a better term, a super yogurt that contains the genetic information of the microbiome. You will learn about the already-proven benefits to our quality of life from the microbiome later in this book.

We warned you that this would seem like science fiction, but as you are about to learn, this is based on hard scientific evidence. Dr. Ruggiero and his colleagues have worked for years in the field of immunotherapy, and they are incredibly excited for the benefits that the feeding of the microbiome can have for support of the immune system. In addition, they believe it can benefit cardiac support, as well as graceful aging.

In essence the realization that the microbiome was in fact a brain, and then furthermore the discovery of how to interact with it, is having very positive effects already on maximizing our quality of life and our ability to live healthy.

As it was recently reported in the American Journal of Clinical Nutrition,

> "Yogurt has been part of the human diet for thousands of years, and during that time a number of health benefits have been associated with its consumption. The goal of the First Global Summit on the Health Effects of Yogurt was to review and evaluate the strength of current scientific knowledge with regard to the health benefits of yogurt and to identify areas where further research is needed. The evidence base for the benefits of yogurt in promoting bone health, maintaining health throughout the life cycle, improving diet quality, and reducing the

incidence of chronic diseases, such as obesity, metabolic syndrome, and cardiovascular disease, was presented."[14]

NOTE: Healthy Yogurts do not reconstitute the Healthy Core Human microbiome

---

However, it has to be clarified here that common yogurts, although beneficial for health, are not designed to reconstitute the healthy core human microbiome. They may contribute to the addition of healthy genetic information, but they are far away from being the "third brain" that has been described above. They do not contain the discovery of the critical combinations of ingredients that do in fact reconstitute the health-core microbiome's genetic makeup.

THE MICROBIOME PROTOCOL™ AND THE MICROBIOME PROTOCOL REGIMEN™

We will also be introducing you to the Microbiome Protocol, which constitutes the microbiome and the Microbiome Protocol Regimen™, comprised of the nutritional components needed to best support the microbiome, the immune system and the other two brains. If you are not convinced yet, perhaps you want to see why the National Institute of Health is allocating more than 150 million dollars to the study of the microbiome.

This is from the NIH website, about the Human Microbiome Project:

---

14. 2014 May; 99(5 Supply):1209S-11S

"In a series of coordinated scientific reports published on June 14, 2012, in Nature and several journals in the Public Library of Science (PLoS), some 200 members of the Human Microbiome Project (HMP) Consortium from nearly 80 universities and scientific institutions report on five years of research. HMP has received $153 million since its launch in fiscal year 2007 from the NIH Common Fund, which invests in high-impact, innovative, trans-NIH research. Individual NIH institutes and centers have provided an additional $20 million in co-funding for HMP consortium research."

"Like 15th century explorers describing the outline of a new continent, HMP researchers employed a new technological strategy to define, for the first time, the normal microbial makeup of the human body," said NIH Director Francis S. Collins, M.D., Ph.D. "HMP created a remarkable reference database by using genome sequencing techniques to detect microbes in healthy volunteers. This lays the foundation for accelerating infectious disease research previously impossible without this community resource."

It is very exciting that NIH is devoting huge sums of money to research around the microbiome.

Dr. Marco Ruggiero and his team, as you will discover, have already demonstrated in their research that the reconstitution of the microbiome can support our immune system, our cardiovascular health, our brain functions, and our overall quality of life.

4

Exciting Published Observational Studies

In this chapter, we are going to introduce you to some amazing work. We will be sharing a collaboration of different peer-reviewed, published studies that have been circulated over the past several years in major scientific journals. We have included some in their original format, while with others, we selected to include the pertinent information to convey the ideas and solutions we are covering in this book. All studies and information shared in this chapter involve the potential to increase the quality of life. This is not just for those facing severe medical challenges; this is to maximize the wellness potential for all of us. Some of the key factors in maximizing the quality of our lives include the following: immune support, heart health support, neurological support, improved circulatory support, and graceful aging support.

EPISTEMOLOGY

The work and studies included in this chapter have been conducted using an epistemological approach. In simple terms, epistemology is the study of the basis or general understanding of knowledge. One definition of epistemology states: Epistemology is the study of the grounds, nature and origins of knowledge and the limits of human understanding. Epistemology deals with the issues such as how knowledge is derived and how it should be tested and validated. Simply put, epistemology works to not only understand *how* something works, but also *why*. The following is an excerpt from an interview I conducted with Dr. Ruggiero discussing the difference in medical testing and theories between double-blind testing and peer-reviewed, published observational studies, and where and how epistemology can play a role.

PETER: We've talked about the published papers. Before speaking with you, I did not comprehend the difference between peer-reviewed observational papers and a double-blind clinical study. Can you address this?

DR. RUGGIERO: Nowadays, in the internet era, there is so much information. But when the information is too much, it risks becoming misinformation. So it's difficult to distinguish between hoax and truth, even though in science, to speak of truth is kind of a philosophical argument. Now, when a researcher – and keep in mind, we prefer to call ourselves researchers rather than scientists – when a researcher makes an observation, whether in the laboratory or in the clinic, we publish these observations in scientific journals. You may be aware of *Science, Nature, The Lancet, The New England Journal of Medicine,* etc. There are dozens of other journals, specializing in cardiology, oncology, and gynecology and so on. So all these journals have this so-called, "peer-review" system. For example, in my laboratory, I make an observation; I put substance "X" in contact with some cancer cells, and I see that this substance kills cancer cells. I say, "Oh! This is interesting!" And I want to share this information with the rest of the medico-scientific community.

I don't put these results of mine on a blog or a website; I send these observations to scientific journals such as *The Journal of Anticancer Research* or *Anticancer Drugs.* Then, they send these results of mine to a panel of experts the most qualified experts in the world in this particular field, who examine my paper and try to reproduce my experiments. They scrutinize my paper to the smallest details. And only after it has passed the review of my peers can this new idea or information be published. Once it is published, then it is listed in search engines like PubMed, which is the database of the National Library of Medicine of the USA, or in Scopus, which is another private database. At that point, this becomes science. So when I say, "It has been scientifically proven that molecule "X" kills cancer cells," I mean that those results have passed the peer-review process.

TWO TYPES OF STUDIES FOR RESEARCH

Going to clinical studies, you essentially have two types of studies. One is the so-called clinical case report (or reports plural), and the other is a double-blind study. The difference is enormous, and we have to be aware of that.

CLINICAL OBSERVATIONS AND CASE REPORTS

The clinical case report could be a single general practitioner in a remote area of Minnesota or Iowa, who sees some notable case, like a person who has a certain disease and uses a certain drug or natural remedy, and the disease gets better or worse (or whatever). And so this general practitioner describes this single clinical case, or maybe two or three clinical cases. Now, because of instant communication and the internet, the medical community all over the world can be aware of these results. Clinical case reports are observations of what works or doesn't work in medicine, done by a single practitioner, or by a small group of practitioners or researchers.

DOUBLE-BLIND STUDIES

Then, you have the double-blind studies. What does this mean? You have to take one thousand or two thousand people, a sizable sample, all of the same gender, same age range, and same type of disease at the same stage, and then you divide them into two or more arms. For one arm, you give them the known treatment; for the other arm, you give them the new drug that you want to test. You have some endpoints. After three months, six months, etc. you make all your calculations, and it's called a "double-blind" study because neither the patient nor the physician knows whether they are giving the old drug or the new drug, or the drug or the placebo during the course of treatment. At the end, you may say, all right, this new drug has X percentage more efficiency than the old one, or less side effects, or whatever. But obviously, to run a double-blind clinical study, you need several institutions, several hospitals; you need an enormous amount of money, and essentially, only big pharmaceutical companies can run these double-blind clinical studies.

DR. RUGGIERO DISCUSSES CLINICAL OBSERVATIONS AND WHY THEY ARE VERY IMPORTANT

As a medical doctor and researcher, I believe that if clinical observations or clinical case reports did not exist, this would be extremely dangerous, because this would mean that the entirety of medical research was only in the hands of big pharma, which could have some serious side effects. But fortunately, scientific papers publish clinical case reports. So what the general practitioner in the remote country town in Iowa has seen could be useful for me in Italy, because I might have a patient with the same identical symptoms, so that information could be extremely useful for me, or for somebody in Japan, or in India. So it is not that double-blind studies have more value than clinical case records. Of course, you have to be smart, and you have to interpret.

PETER: So without a double-blind peer-reviewed study, no drug comes on the market, right? Let's say your observational study, this clinical practitioner study that you found was conducted in Iowa, and you used it on one of your patients. Isn't there a risk there? Especially with big pharma's endless reach and limitless funds?

DR. RUGGIERO: Absolutely. And as I told you, I've been in the big pharma industry for years, and the point is that if they don't like the results, they don't publish them. They simply pretend that they have not done those double-blind clinical studies. But, unfortunately, double-blind clinical studies are not a guarantee for safety. Do you remember the Viox ordeal?

Thousands of deaths occurred due to the drug, simply because its manufacturers missed something that was obvious to those who had studied the field and similar drugs for the previous twenty years. And Viox was approved after phase one, phase two, and phase three of the clinical trials. So it had undergone all possible scrutiny, and nevertheless, we're talking about thousands of deaths. So this tells you that a double-blind clinical study is not a guarantee at all. I don't know how many people have died as a consequence of clinical case reports, but I know that thousands of people died in that specific case, and we may even say that they were killed by those double-blind clinical studies.

PETER: Well, for the purpose of this show, what I wanted people to understand is that an observational clinical study, just so I'm clear, can also give a doctor enough confidence to perhaps apply these protocols, especially if they're natural, they're not a drug per se. Is that correct, that this gives them *way* more assurance than just if Joe Shmoe and I are in our kitchen and mix up some rhubarb and whatever and say, "Hey, this is going to make your headaches go away," or something, right?

DR. RUGGIERO: Yes. You are absolutely right, because even if it is the observation of only one case, nevertheless it is so well documented that it has gone through the peer-review process. So even if it is only one case, you know the famous black swan of Aristotle's logic. You may say, "All swans are white," because all swans look white. But if you see only one black swan, it doesn't matter if it's only one; one is sufficient to make your statement false, as they say in philosophy.

So let's say you have pancreatic cancer, which today is considered the deadliest of all cancers. And then you have this general practitioner in a remote country town who says, "I have this pancreatic cancer patient. I have treated this patient with whatever, and he has been cured. And I can document this reliably." Up to that point, this case report is accepted by the peer-review system. So what it tells us for the thousands of pancreatic cancer patients all over the world is that their disease can be cured. That is the black swan. It is important that it is well documented. If it weren't well documented, it would not have been accepted for publication.

DR. MARCO RUGGIERO WROTE THE FOLLOWING PORTION OF THIS CHAPTER.

The studies discussed are primarily Dr. Ruggiero's personal work, which was peer reviewed and published in a number of different major medical journals. Dr. Ruggiero has been overly gracious to take time from his busy schedule to provide insight into his life's work to give you, the reader, direct insight into this incredible information. We are eternally grateful for him. All studies and articles mentioned can be found through the citations or through the PubMed website.

IMMUNE SUPPORT TO MAXIMIZE
OUR WELLNESS POTENTIAL

When I began working on the microbiome, I knew that it contained all the information that is required to live long, healthy lives, because the microbiome contains 99% of all the genetic information that we need. Being the complex ecosystem that it is, it can be compared to the pluvial forest of Amazonia, which contain plants that produce substances from which all the drugs to heal mankind can be distilled. In the wealth of information of the healthy microbiome, there is all we need to enable the correct development and function of our organs and to even improve their performances without running the risk of exhausting them.

VITAMIN D AXIS WAS STUDIED
FOR THE PAST 20 YEARS

For the past 20 years, I focused my research on a particular signaling pathway that, until recently, was not considered a part of the microbiome. I am referring to the vitamin D axis, a complex metabolic pathway comprised of vitamin D in its various forms (vitamin D2 and D3 for example), its intracellular receptor termed vitamin D receptor (VDR), and the carrier protein that is aptly designated vitamin D-binding protein (VDBP, also designated Gc protein). My contribution to the research on the vitamin D axis was recognized by the Editors of the prestigious scientific journal Kidney International, a journal of the Nature Publishing Group, when, in 2009, they invited me to write a review on the most-discussed aspect surrounding this topic, namely: "which is the best dosage of vitamin D?" Accordingly, my invited commentary was entitled "Chronic kidney disease and vitamin D: how much is adequate?"[15]

Vitamin D has been known for years for its role in calcium metabolism and, therefore, in preventing rickets and osteoporosis. More recently however, it was discovered that it plays crucial roles in the development and function of our immune system and our first and second brains. A search for "vitamin D and immune system" in PubMed yields more than 3,000 peer-reviewed papers, and a search for "vitamin D and brain" yields more than 1,000 such papers. Vitamin D and its deficiencies, have been involved in practically all human diseases ranging from cancer (more than 8,000 papers) to autism, with studies demonstrating that vitamin D supplementation leads to improvement of the core symptoms of autism (*Core symptoms of autism improved after vitamin D supplementation.*)[16]

My scientific contribution to vitamin D research was in studying the role of the other two components of the vitamin D axis: the VDR and the VDBP. In fact, vitamin D cannot exert its effects without these two proteins that actually translate the vitamin D signal into a language that can be understood by the cells, a signal that, thanks to the interactions between the VDBP and the VDR ultimately leads to significant changes in the DNA of the cell. A great number of genes are turned on and an equally great number of genes are turned off thanks to the interconnected signaling passing through the VDBP and the VDR. In simpler words, these two proteins, the VDBP and

15. *Kidney Int.* 2009 Nov; 76(9):931-3

16. Jia F, Wang B, Shan L, Xu Z, Staal WG, Du L. *Pediatrics.* 2015 Jan; 135(1):e196-8

the VDR, in mediating the signal of vitamin D, profoundly affect the behavior of cellular DNA, protecting us from most, if not all, diseases.

It appears that vitamin D has played a primary role in the evolution of all species and of the human species in particular, up to the point that a paper in PubMed is aptly entitled: *"Does vitamin D make the world go 'round'?"* It is not a coincidence that this paper was published in a journal entitled *Breastfeeding Medicine,* a journal dedicated to a food, mother's milk, that is the starting point for the building of the microbiome.[17]

According to this publication:

> "Vitamin D has emerged from obscurity, and its effects on various organ systems throughout the body down to the cellular level are being discovered. What was once thought to be a simple hormone affecting only bone and calcium metabolism has shifted. We no longer see vitamin D as a "vitamin" important only in childhood, but as a complex hormone that is involved not only in calcium homeostasis but also in the integrity of the innate immune system. Vitamin D deficiency is linked to inflammatory and long-latency diseases such as multiple sclerosis, rheumatoid arthritis, tuberculosis, diabetes, and various cancers, to name a few."

In fact, vitamin D is much more than a "vitamin". It is a hormone, a secosteroid hormone to be precise, and it affects the functioning of the most important genes that control practically all our cellular functions.

---

17. 2008 Dec; 3(4):239-50

When the authors of the paper "Does Vitamin D Make the World Go Round?" wrote their article in 2008, however, they were unaware of the role of the microbiome in the metabolism of vitamin D, and therefore, they only referred to mother's milk as a nutrient rather than the source of the most fundamental information. Now, we know that the interaction between mother's milk and the microbes in the intestine involves the metabolism of at least one of the components of the vitamin D axis, the VDBP, a protein that has been the main focus of my research since 2009.

The VDBP, or Gc protein, is a multifunctional carrier protein that exerts a number of functions in health and disease, and I wrote a seminal article on this issue in a specialized journal, European Nephrology, in 2011.[18] What is most interesting, however, is that VDBP, in addition to performing a number of biological functions, is also the precursor of another protein that has powerful effects on the immune system as well as on the brain.

This latter protein has a designation that is almost impossible to pronounce, "N-Acetylgalactosamine-glycosylated vitamin D binding protein", and therefore, for the sake of clarity, it's abbreviated to NAG (from the first letters of N-Acetyl and Galactosamine) or GcMAF (since it derives from the Gc protein). It is also worth noting that the stem of the name "Galactosamine" refers to milk, since galactose is the carbohydrate of milk, from the ancient Greek *galakt*. The GcMAF protein is a derivative of VDBP, and it is formed in our plasma every time that there is an immune response. We discovered that this protein

---

18. Ruggiero, M., Pacini, S.: *The vitamin D axis in chronic kidney disease: state of the art and future perspectives. European Nephrology*. 5: 15-9 2011).

not only activates the cells of the immune system, but that it also directly inhibits the growth of cancer cells, and it showed interesting neuroprotective effects that can be exploited in the prevention and cure of a number of neurological and neurodevelopmental disorders ranging from Alzheimer's to autism.[19]

GCMAF PROTEIN FUNDAMENTALLY IMPORTANT TO THE MICROBIOME

In addition, we discovered that the protein GcMAF is formed in our intestine, thanks to the action of the microbiome upon its precursor, the VDBP, or Gc protein, and therefore, it exerts a fundamental role in the development and function of the third brain as well as the immune system. Therefore, it was not a surprise when we discovered that the third brain recreated in a cup contained a lot of this active GcMAF protein that was naturally formed by the action of the microbiome on milk and colostrum.

As we have described in other chapters, the engineering of the healthy human core microbiome, in the form of a super food, brings with it innumerable consequences as far as maintaining health and our quality of life are concerned. Here, I wish to describe a few that are directly connected to the presence of this GcMAF protein, a member of the vitamin D axis around which, apparently, the world revolves, or at least the biological world.

The GcMAF protein, in combination with the VDR and healthy fatty acids, such as the oleic acid that is found in olives and olive oil, exerts a number of effects at the level of the human DNA that

---

19. *J Neurosci Res.* 2015 Mar 18. *Anticancer Drugs.* 2015 Feb; 26(2):197-209.

further highlight the importance of the cross-talk between the micro-biome and the human genome. In fact, the active GcMAF, a product of the genetic information contained in the microbiome and this microbe-derived information, interacts and modifies the information contained in the human DNA.

OUR MAJOR BREAKTHROUGH: WE FORMULATED "A FOOD FOR YOUR THIRD BRAIN"

After hundreds of experiments, we finally discovered that the genetic information contained in the human microbiome could be reconstituted in a super food we were able to formulate. We call this new super food a dessert cup. To our delight, this new super food positively influenced the production of energy at the level of the mitochondria in the heart. It is worth noting, however, that very recent, yet unpublished, studies seem to indicate that the GcMAF protein acts like a carrier. In other words, it is the sort of vehicle that delivers molecules with powerful biological actions to their cell tar-gets. Among the bioactive molecules carried by GcMAF, of particular importance are vitamins of the D group, fatty acids such as oleic acid, and glycosaminoglycans, which are sugar-based molecules that exert a fundamental role in cell-to-cell signaling.

OBSERVATION STUDY FOR
HEALTHY HEART SUPPORT

The heart beats incessantly from the time it is formed in the womb until we die, and unlike skeletal muscles that need minutes or hours to recover after an effort, the heart only has a few milliseconds to recover between each beat. In those milliseconds, it has to rebuild the energy in those power plants of the cell: the mitochondria. Just as happens in trained athletes, whose skeletal muscle recovery is faster and more efficient than in sedentary people, a trained heart in good health shows a faster and more efficient recovery compared with a heart in less-than-perfect conditions. It is possible to measure this little time that serves for cardiac recovery, which is called Iso-Volumetric Relaxation Time or IVRT.

Having a good practical expertise in ultrasonography, I was able to easily measure my basal IVRT, which luckily was within the normal range. Then, I extracted the information contained in the third brain and re-created it in the form of a creamy dessert. I consumed this creamy concoction, (recipe to follow in upcoming chapter. Make sure to read on) and quite amazingly, my IVRT significantly diminished, thus indicating a sudden improvement in the efficiency of energy production in the mitochondria of my heart. In a more structured series of experiments, we compared these effects *in vivo* with those obtained *in vitro* using an appropriate reconstitution of the vitamin D axis, and our results were so convincing as to be accepted for publication in a special issue of the scientific Journal *Nutrients*, dedicated to the description of the novel effects of vitamin D.[20]

OUR NUTRITIONAL DISCOVERY SUPPORTS HEART HEALTH: CARDIOVASCULAR SUPPORT FOR DESSERT

In this paper we hypothesized that vitamin D, its receptor (the VDR) and the GcMAF carrier protein could play a significant role in the prevention of cardiovascular diseases, as clearly stated in the title of the study. However, a more general consequence of our study lies in the possibility to support cardiac health through the third brain produced as a delicious dessert or healthy snack. And this possibility further reinforces the concept that food is not only calories and nutrients, but more importantly, genetic information that interacts with the functioning of our genes.

In another set of studies that were published very recently and are listed in PubMed, we discovered another property of this active GcMAF protein that is directly related to the role of the microbiome in the development and function of the brain, and it could not be different, since the microbiome is the third brain.

20. *Effects of vitamin D3 and paricalcitol on immature cardiomyocytes: a novel role for vitamin D analogs in the prevention of cardiovascular diseases.* Pacini S, Morucci G, Branca JJ, Aterini S, Amato M, Gulisano M, Ruggiero M. *Nutrients.* 2013 Jun 7; 5(6):2076-92

NEURON SUPPORT FOR NEURONS AND GLIAL CELLS

Since I have dedicated a great part of my academic career to the study of oncology, it was almost unavoidable that these observations were born out of our interest in cancer therapies. We were particularly interested in the effects of a platinum derivative, oxaliplatin, a very efficient chemotherapeutic drug that is successfully used in a number of cancers. Regrettably, however, this drug shows a severe side effect: the onset of an excruciating neuropathic pain that leads to severe dysfunction. This side effect may be so severe that patients prefer not to adhere to the therapeutic regime and rather incur the risk of a progression of the disease.

In our two studies, published very recently, we demonstrate that the information contained in the microbiome, and more specifically, in the carrier protein GcMAF, is able to counteract the damage inflicted by oxaliplatin to human neurons and glial cells.[21]

We performed experiments in vitro where we challenged human neurons and glial cells with oxaliplatin, and we recorded the cell damage in terms of decreased energy production and reduction of the connections between cells. As is described in other parts of this book, the interconnections between neurons and glial cells in our brains are at the basis of the functioning of our minds. Then, we performed the same experiments having pre-treated the cells with the GcMAF protein, the same one that we can find in the third brain in the dessert cup. In other words, we put the cells in culture in the same situation of a subject who first drinks the third brain in a dessert cup and, 24 hours later, is treated with platinum-based chemotherapy.

---

21. *J Neurosci Res.* 2015 Mar 18. *Anticancer Drugs.* 2015 Feb; 26(2):197-209.

We observed that the GcMAF protein protected both neurons and glial cells from the damage inflicted by platinum (a heavy metal). Being experts in molecular biology, we also elucidated the molecular mechanism responsible for such a protective effect; the active GcMAF protein instructed the DNA of the cells to turn on the gene coding for a factor termed VEGF that is responsible for the repair of the damages inflicted to the neurons and the glial cells. And more interestingly, the consequences that these observation bear are that this VEGF is not specific for platinum-induced damages, but for all type of damages that can be inflicted to human neurons and glial cells by all types of toxicants, as well as by aging.

In other words, even though our objective in performing those experiments was simply to ameliorate the side effects of a particular form of chemotherapy, we had found a way to counteract aging and to protect the brain inside our heads thanks to the third brain that, once more, proved its incommensurable importance.

In fact, from our studies, it emerges that the information contained in the microbiome under the form of the GcMAF protein, produced by the microbes fermenting mother's milk, interacts with the information encoded in the human DNA, thus stimulating the human DNA to produce a factor, the VEGF, that is essential in the development of the brain and in repairing all types of damage to the brain.

SUPPORT FOR GRACEFUL AGING AND NEURON PROTECTION

It is evident that the applications of these observations are impressive, since we now have the way to protect our first brain by reconstituting the third brain simply with a food. And this could find applications not only in the field of heavy metal-related toxicity but also, and probably more importantly, in the field of anti-aging.

In fact, we have demonstrated that the proteins produced by the microbiome not only protect our neurons, but they actually instruct our neurons to make new connections, thus forming new neural circuits. We can create new thoughts, new concepts and new memories. The support of the healthy microbiome helps us to have more neural webs of interconnections.

> **NOTE:** Again, I want to emphasize that we are not in any way replacing traditional medical approaches with this nutritional discovery. Our discovery in no way cures or treats any disease, period. We offer our observations as additional information that can be complimentary and supportive of traditional and clinically proven medical protocols.

Our goal and our observations support our approach to maximizing the wellness potential and quality of life for all of us. None of these statements have been evaluated by the FDA. In no way should you interpret this as a substitute for sound medical advice. As always, it is recommended that you check with your medical doctor before embarking on any nutritional approach.

5

Evaluating a Patient's Health

When Dr. Ruggiero sees patients, like most physicians, he puts together a program that provides him with a ground-level evaluation of each individual he is working with. Not only is this used to get a feel for the patient, it is also used to provide the patient with a protocol to follow to maximize their current state of health. The very first thing that Dr. Ruggiero does when evaluating a patient's health is to evaluate their nutritional history.

Dr. Ruggiero and his clinicians spend several hours analyzing each patient's eating habits. As Dr. Ruggiero has said, there is no therapy, surgery, drug, or procedure that can overcome poor nutritional habits. It may also be important to state that some of these individuals may have thought they were eating "clean", but they fail to have the proper nutritional needs and protein/carbohydrate/fat ratio that is needed to optimize their potential to achieve optimal health. The following text was written by Dr. Ruggiero, describing the steps taken and why they are addressed.

REBALANCING THE BODY'S NUTRIENTS

First of all, it is fundamental to remember that food is not only calories and nutrients. It is the vastly more important genetic information that interacts with our DNA. The concept of calories in food was introduced more than 100 years ago when it was (very wrongly) supposed that the human body was like a steam engine and functioned by burning different types of combustibles, such as proteins, fats and sugars. Nothing was known at that time of the genetic information in DNA, and even less of the microbiome and the complex interactions between these types of information.

Now that we know much more about the true significance of food, we can understand why even in well-nourished or seemingly over-nourished people, some essential nutrients may be missing. In fact, nutrients are not just those that provide calories; nutrients are also those that provide the genetic information that allows the microbiome to interact with our genes in a marvelously complex web of interconnections. To function properly, our microbiome needs the appropriate food and essential nutrients. The microbiome needs these essential nutrients that may have gone missing from our bodies. Unfortunately, many of these essential nutrients that are required to form the microbiome as well as the human parts of our bodies have been drained, corrupted, or destroyed by modern farming and food production. The good news is, they can be found.

My search for immune-stimulating proteins and carrier proteins such as vitamin-D binding proteins led me to discover that we can recreate and actually produce them in a kitchen. Rebalancing nutrition is a very difficult task. It is, however, relatively simple at times to prescribe a specific, appropriate drug for a specific disease. It can take countless hours to determine nutritional deficiencies or the nutritional needs of a given patient, in particular when dealing with the deficiencies of the microbiome.

I believe in a holistic nutritional approach to the health of a patient as the very first step we must take. This is not as a replacement for medical procedures. It is used in conjunction with them to provide the best possible quality of life as long as possible for all my patients.

MOST PEOPLE ARE SEVERELY LACKING IN SUFFICIENT NUTRITIONAL BALANCE

Most people do not have anything even close to balanced and sufficient nutrition in their lives. This makes rebalancing their bodies that much more difficult. No medical therapy, no matter how effective, will work 100% of the time if nutrition is not attended to first. Now that we understand that nutrition is much more than burning logs to produce heat (i.e. much more than calories), it is easy to conceive that without a proper and consistent supply of the correct genetic information through food, our genes cannot work as they are supposed to, and hence, all types of diseases may arise.

THE INITIAL CONSULTATION

The first thing I do when assessing a patient is look at their nutritional status from this new perspective based upon the research on the microbiome. We have learned that imbalances in the microbiome are often associated with systemic inflammation. Inflammation is the basis of all chronic diseases, and therefore, one of the first things to look at is the degree of inflammation they are suffering. We utilize an inexpensive and simple tool called the Prognostic Inflammatory and Nutritional Index (PINI) to analyze a patient's level of inflammation. This score gives us a baseline from which to begin rebalancing that patient's nutrition. In cancer, as well as in other chronic diseases, you cannot produce enough natural defense molecules, which are the cancer-fighting proteins in your body. This is because there are enzymes, produced either by viruses or by cancer cells, that destroy the precursors to these proteins. One means of combating this is by introducing proteins from outside the body through a food supplement or an immuno-therapeutic drug. In most cases, a food supplement is preferable, because it is more natural and more efficient.

EPIGENETICS: TAKING CONTROL OF YOUR DNA

We rebalance nutrition as a method of combating the negative effects of the environment on the body. We are bombarded with toxins, free radicals, viruses, infections, parasites; you name it, and it's out there. We know that the cause of cancer is not one single mutation, but rather a complex interaction between mutations in our DNA and the so-called epi-mutations that pertain to the realm of epigenetics. The realm of epigenetics essentially is the interaction between the environment and our DNA and the way the information in our DNA is "read". The genetic information in the environment is obviously of utmost importance in these interactions. The environment is essential to this process. We can do little against mutations, although if we were exposed to less smoking, less ionizing radiation, fewer mutagenic chemicals, and so on, we would be better off.

But mutations can and do happen spontaneously and honestly; there is little we can do about it. What we can do is avoid the expression, the manifestation of these mutations. We can minimize, if not eradicate, the effects of those mutations. This new field of science is called epigenetics, or epigenomics, where "epi," derived from ancient Greek, refers to something that is above DNA. To make a complex matter simple, genetics is the study of the information encoded in DNA. Epigenetics is the study of how this information is interpreted by the cell. It is like a text. Take Dante's *Comedy*; you can study the sequence of the letters in the text and the meaning of each word, and this is comparable to genetics. Then, you can study the meaning of the entire *Comedy*, the journey of Dante and Virgil from Hell to Heaven, the allegory, what Dante wanted to say, how we interpret his work in modern times and so on, and this is epigenetic. Sometimes, the information in our DNA is corrupted, mutated, and there is little if anything that we can do to fix a mutation.

But, using the knowledge that we have acquired on the epigenome, we can work at the level of proper nutrition and appropriate lifestyle to allow us to *control* our genetic information, which is how our cells interpret the genetic information.

MAKING WAR ON CANCEROUS CELLS

If the cancer cells could not fool our immune system, cancer simply would not exist, because our immune system is very well equipped to kill cancer cells right away. From a statistical point of view, we have cancer cells in our body from the moment we are born or even before. Our bodies prevent us from accumulating cancer cells by eliminating those cells throughout our lives. Our immune system, most of the time, recognizes these foreign enemy cells and induces *apoptosis*, their physiological death. But cancer cells also follow the rules of evolution, or we would not have cancer cells at all. If cancer did not evolve to disguise itself, it would be eradicated. But it does evolve, and as it does, like a foreign enemy wearing the uniform of those it is invading, it hides in our bodies and perpetrates its crimes while the immune system fails to see and react to the threat.

This is where epigenetics and immunotherapy comes into play. Through supplying and restoring the healthy microbiome, we equip the immune system to recognize those cancer cells disguised as normal cells. Or, to be more precise, the microbiome *is* an essential part of the immune system, and here we could think of food that restores the microbiome as a daily transplant of a healthy immune system.

It is as if we are equipping our body's soldiers with scanners that allow them to detect the hidden enemy. The nutritional immunotherapy approach thus involves empowering the immune system to discover, attack, and kill cancer cells. It is very different than the traditional chemotherapy approach, even though, in many cases, the two approaches can be applied together with a positive synergistic effect. For example, as previously described, we recently published two peer-reviewed papers that are listed in PubMed, demonstrating that certain molecules pertaining to this nutritional immunotherapeutic approach have counteracted the side effects of a powerful chemotherapeutic agent, a platinum derivative, with the potential of improving the overall anti-cancer effect of this type of chemothera-py.[22] In fact, if the epigenetic approach is like equipping your soldiers with scanners, the chemotherapy approach is equivalent to lobbing bombs indiscriminately about the battlefield, killing both your own forces and the enemy's. Chemotherapy kills everything, both the good and the bad, and sometimes kills more good than it does bad. However, as the papers quoted above demonstrate, the nutritional immunotherapeutic approach based on epigenetics can direct those bombs toward the enemy, making them "intelligent" and at the same time providing a shield for your own forces.

IMMUNOTHERAPEUTIC APPROACH SPECIFICALLY TARGETS

This immunotherapeutic approach is extremely targeted by definition, because it employs the most sophisticated defense system that nature gave us—the immune system. We propose that we don't kill the cancer cells with an external agent. We instead propose to boost the immune system and empower *it* to kill the cancer cells from within, by employing a precision we could never hope to achieve from outside the body.

This method works to support the effectiveness of chemotherapy and radiation as an additional tool to improve the quality of life of patients. In no way does it replace the need and use of chemotherapy,

---

22. *Effects of oxaliplatin and oleic acid Gc-protein-derived macrophage-activating factor on murine and human microglia.* Branca JJ, Morucci G, Malentacchi F, Gelmini S, Ruggiero M, Pacini S. *J Neurosci Res.* 2015 Mar 18.
Gc-protein-derived macrophage activating factor counteracts the neuronal damage induced by oxaliplatin. Morucci G, Branca JJ, Gulisano M, Ruggiero M, Paternostro F, Pacini A, Di Cesare Mannelli L, Pacini S. *Anticancer Drugs.* 2015 Feb; 26(2):197-209.

radiation or surgery. On the contrary, in many instances it makes surgery or radiation therapy possible so that the patient can receive the greatest benefit from both approaches. We in no way want a patient to think we are offering a cure for any disease. Our goal is to support the patient's quality of life by providing support to the function of the immune system through food for your microbiome (third brain).

The change in nutritional lifestyle support and quality of life has been documented in just a few of the peer-reviewed studies in chapter four. These studies illustrate the benefits of maximizing wellness potential and quality of life for everyday people, not just for those facing severe medical challenges.

Some of the key factors in maximizing the quality of our lives are the following:

- Heart Health Support
- Graceful Aging Support
- Neurological Support
- Immune Support
- Circulation Support

Dr. Ruggiero has spent three decades forensically researching methods to fine-tune the inner workings of our immune system. That is why the initial dietary analysis is critical to the process of maximizing wellness. He needs to see where the patients are starting and create protocols or regimens to best suit their needs. Dr. Ruggiero is insistent that the patients follow the Microbiome Protocol™ and the Microbiome Protocol Regimen™ as he has laid it out as closely as possible. With his patients, he will create individualized plans, but he confidently knows that the framework of the Microbiome Protocol and Regimen has enhanced and may continue to enhance the quality of life for his pateints, friends and colleagues, regardless of their health situations

I WAS THERE FOR A PATIENT EVALUATION

With patient consent, I was privileged and fortunate to have observed Dr. Ruggiero and his team at work. It was a quite remarkable experience, as documented below.

Dr. Ruggiero often spends a considerable amount of time interviewing his patients. I had the privilege to witness a few of his initial evaluations, with patient permission. His bedside manner was impeccable, making his patients feel at ease with his warm manner. Dr. Ruggiero interviews and documents specific information regarding his patients' lifestyles, dietary habits, previous diagnoses, and treatments, as well as any other important information. He often spends well over an hour gathering this critical information.

During one of my observations, Dr. Ruggiero, his patient, and a team of doctors were present. He carefully conducted his interview, and upon completion, Dr. Ruggiero, also a highly skilled radiologist, performed a non-invasive ultrasonography for further assessment.

Dr. Ruggiero deemed (from his assessment) that this patient had a particularly sluggish immune system. I witnessed the actual sonography of the patient's spleen. Utilizing this information, Dr. Ruggiero wanted to demonstrate the effect of utilizing a component of The Microbiome Protocol, the Bravo probiotic. We looked at the spleen before and after consumption of Bravo. After consumption, the Doppler ultrasonography showed amazing activity— displaying brilliant colors of red, yellow, and blue. Dr. Ruggiero explained that the colorful display was in fact the immune system lighting up. Dr. Ruggiero calmly said, "Well, the macrophages are going to work and the immune system is now being supported".

He was quick to caution that this was not evidence of any type of a cure. It was more a great indication that there was now enhanced observable activity in the patient's immune system. The patient continued conventional treatments with the team of doctors as prescribed. After she followed Dr. Ruggiero's Microbiome Protocol and Microbiome Protocol Regimen for five months, we are happy to report that her quality of life has drastically improved.

This experience was unforgettable, as I was able to see this truly groundbreaking technology first hand.

PREVENTATIVE INTERVENTION IS A GREAT STRATEGY

In my last book, *TDOS Syndrome and Solutions*, I referenced experts who stated that we need to be looking for more preventative, interventional approaches to maximize our wellness potential. At the time *TDOS* was written, we did not have knowledge of Dr. Ruggiero or his discovery of The Microbiome Protocol and Regimen.

Upon meeting Dr. Ruggiero and learning about The Microbiome Protocol and The Microbiome Protocol Regimen, I have been able to support my own immune system utilizing this great interventional tool. This makes sense to me—to do everything possible to support my immune system and to give myself the greatest preventative strategy to achieve the best quality of life for as long as possible.

Please note that Dr. Ruggiero is not making any claims of curing any diseases. He is simply stating his observations with patients that have, in many cases, increased the quality of their lives. This is a noble goal for any health professional.

As we stated before, The Microbiome Protocol and Regimen are not substitutes for conventional medical procedures or protocols, but are being used in conjunction with established and proven medical procedures and protocols in cooperation with the patients' medical doctors.

It is our recommendation that you consult with your health professional, as it is always the best advice before embarking on any new nutritional approach such as The Microbiome Protocol or The Microbiome Regimen.

SECTION II

Rebalancing the Body's Nutrients and Food for Your Three Brains

An integral part of "The New Health Conversation" is to not only provide our readers with the latest information regarding health and wellness, but also to provide answers and solutions. There seem to be myriad books addressing the current state of affairs in the health industry, but few provide solutions. What good is a problem without a solution? We are fortunate that Dr. Ruggiero not only broke ground identifying the third brain, but also reverse-engineered it to find a way to feed it.

This section will cover different foods and solutions to feed all three brains in the body. It only makes sense that nutrition plays a major part in healing the body. The main purpose of providing the body with the proper foods, vitamins and minerals is to give the human body the best shot at staving off illness. Chapter 11 covers the age-old practice of immunotherapy, which basically boosts the body's natural defense system to fight sickness. We are also fortunate to hear the stories from Dr. Ruggiero himself of how he came to discover "The Dessert Cup".

The information in the first section of this book is significant enough to change the path of human beings. We feel we are on the verge of a drastic shift in how we view human science. As important as that information is, it would have much less of an impact without the following section. The following information could drastically change the health and wellness world for the better.

6

Food for Your First Brain

My good friend and colleague, Dr. John Gray, the author of *Men Are from Mars, Women Are from Venus,* was the first researcher to introduce me to the concept of food for the brain, in our heads, over a decade ago. It really hit home for me in 2003 and helped me create the fascinating curiosity that still drives me for answers today.

John helped my youngest son Colin, who I wrote about in *TDOS Syndrome and Solution,* and in the preface in his new book, *Staying Focused in a Hyper World.* Colin suffered from extreme challenges such as lack of concentration, anxiety and depression. I want to thank John Gray again for helping Colin to greatly improve his quality of life. Colin was able to eliminate the medications he was taking more than a decade ago and has lived a much happier and healthier life as a result. John made me aware of natural supplements and minerals that are in very short supply or non-existent in our current food supplies. These foods and supplements are critically important as food for the first brain.

We have asked the following question as part of "The New Health Conversation":

Is your food doing something to you, or, is your food doing something for you?

This question has become even more important as our co-author brilliantly stated that food is not only made of carbohydrates, fats and protein.

For many of us foodies in the world, food serves not just to give us pleasure, to fill our bellies or even to provide us fuel for our daily activities. Dr. Ruggiero has shed light on the most critical importance of food: as the communicator of genetic information to our genes. Food is the main carrier of critical genetic information to our genes, which in turn tell our cells what to do. If it communicates incomplete or corrupted genetic information to our genes, then the genes will in turn communicate incomplete and corrupted information to our cells. The cells react to this bad genetic information in many horrific ways, including replicating and creating cellular mutations. That, then, becomes the root of many of the out-of-control health challenges we face as a world today.

Does it make sense that corrupted and incomplete genetic information passed along to our first brain is a huge limiting factor in giving us the highest possible quality of life? The brain in our heads, as you have learned, is just one of three operating systems for the human body. Just like the programs that make computers function, it is the software, not the hardware, that makes the computer carry out its tasks. When our computers get corrupted information through viruses or worn-out software, the computers start to fail. They become sluggish at first and then continue to deteriorate to the point where they become literally useless unless we fix the corrupted software.

Is it any wonder that unless we provide our brains with uncorrupted, high-quality genetic information, we become stressed out and foggy headed? Are we maximizing our quality of life and wellness potential? We need very specific foods to carry the best and most uncorrupted genetic information to our brains if we are to live at our highest quality of life.

It is important that we share our research for the best foods for your first brain, in order to maximize your brain's highest potential. The following research has been passed on by Dr. John Gray. We are so grateful to him for his willingness to share this with us.

"There is not a one solution fits all, but you will learn what supplements work and why they do. You will learn what food to eat and what to avoid. You will gain the insight you and your children need to achieve optimal brain function and focus. I do not know what is right for you, but I can share the missing insight for you to discover what will work for you. When taking supplements, it is important to see them not as drugs with dangerous side effects but as the missing ingredients from the food we eat. Just as you might add a long list of spices to make a meal more tasty and healthy, you can now add a list of supplements to make it more nutritious. Here are supplements and foods that promote healthy brain function." John Gray, PhD, author of *Men Are from Mars, Women Are from Venus.*

These are the foods and enhanced foods that have been identified by numerous experts to give the brain what it requires to work at optimum levels. Dr. John Gray has specifically targeted the following nutrients and minerals to feed the cranial brain in order to maximize wellness.

VITAMIN C

Hands down, vitamin C is the most important vitamin for the brain. In order for the best absorption to occur, our liver needs to produce glutathione. To make glutathione, we need a healthy, drug-free liver, and we need to consume foods high in cysteine. Cysteine is an amino acid that helps the body produce glutathione. Glutathione activates vitamin C and assists the body in detoxifying the toxic chemicals and heavy metals that interfere with body and brain function.

The standard American diet is extremely high in added sugars and simple carbohydrates, including favorites like white rice, traditional sandwich bread, chips, cookies, and cakes made from processed flour. These foods spike blood sugar levels, and thus deplete the body of vitamin C. The result: a lifetime of gradual injury to the brain.

As you will learn, a major component of Dr. Ruggiero's work with patients with major health challenges begins by drastically lowering sugar and carbohydrate intake in their daily diets. He recommends consumption of approximately 20% carbohydrates daily for those with compromised immunity. This shift toward a ketogenic-like diet is the cornerstone of his work. For an individual who does not have a compromised immune system, weight loss may be welcomed. It is important to state that an individual does not want to lose lean muscle mass. This is why it is critical to have the highest quality of bio-available protein available.

PRISTINE PROTEIN POWDERS

Not all proteins are created equal. This statement reminds me of the old joke: What do you call the doctor who graduates last in the class? Or who passes the boards by one question?

You call him Doctor.

When searching for the correct proteins to nourish the body— it is no different.

Many grocery stores, vitamin shops, or big-box warehouses are packed with a variety of protein drinks and powders. How do you choose?

WHAT THE EXPERTS ARE SAYING ABOUT PROTEIN

In several of John Gray's books, he specifically recommends Super Food Shakes from New Zealand and Australia. He has chosen these shakes because they are made with an undenatured whey protein. These are the very same shakes referenced in the other books in "The New Health Conversation" series. For individuals with whey or milk allergies (not lactose-intolerance), there is a plant-based (non-soy) alternative that mimics the bioavailability of these Super Shakes.

I recently had the honor of interviewing Dr. Colgan on my television program, "The New Health Conversation", on PBS Rocky Mountain. Michael Colgan, PhD, is one of the world's leading experts on protein. Colgan and his research team have analyzed nearly every protein source on the planet, including animal, plant, and even sea-weed. Dr. Colgan has made it clear that after researching proteins for more than 30 years, he has discovered that proteins are incredibly complex substances and are not all the same. Some protein sources are much healthier and supply more usable protein than others. His conclusion: Whey protein from New Zealand or Australia's grass-fed dairy cows are the best protein options in the world. His reasonings are stated below.

PROTEIN VITALLY IMPORTANT TO OUR BODIES

You may be surprised to learn that our bodies are made up of over 350,000 different kinds of proteins, some of them formed in amino acid chains over 30,000 units in length. This means that to be healthy and full of vitality, we need to consume protein sources that provide everything we need. Colgan believes that protein may be the single most important nutrient, and many of us are simply not getting enough of it. I want to emphasize again that the proteins in our body are incredibly complex and vitally important to our health and well-being. In short, any high heat processing (as used in most pasteurization processes in North America) of proteins causes them to be denatured, which means the natural protein folds break down. Why is the breaking down of the protein folds as a result of high pasteurization or cooking so detrimental to the effectiveness of the protein? Whey protein reduces oxidative stress.

> "When considering the antioxidant-boosting properties of whey protein, quality counts. There is evidence that the undenatured form of whey is superior to the denatured form. Unlike denatured whey protein, which is broken into individual amino acids, undenatured whey protein is carefully processed so that the natural folds within the protein are maintained. Undenatured whey protein has

been shown to have greater antioxidant-boosting and also immune-enhancing abilities than denatured protein.

Oxidative stress is a major cause of biological aging and occurs when the body's antioxidant systems are overwhelmed by the amount of harmful oxidative agents. These oxidative agents cause damage to cells and are created as a result of environmental, dietary, and psychological stress, as well as from the normal processes of metabolism. Glutathione is an important antioxidant that guards cells from injury that contributes to aging, and whey protein is a potent supplier of the building blocks of glutathione.

The ability of whey protein to boost glutathione synthesis is of particular importance to older people, whose ability to make glutathione decreases with age. By their sixties and seventies, some elderly people have been shown to have glutathione levels 50 percent lower than adults in their twenties and thirties. By increasing glutathione levels in older people, whey protein helps fight oxidative stress and delays the progression of cellular aging."[23]

Why are these experts choosing proteins from New Zealand and Australia?

Can't we get an undenatured protein in the US?

Why grass-fed? The cattle in New Zealand and Australia are grass-fed and are not given antibiotics or hormones. Cows are meant to eat grass freely in a pasture. In the United States, most of the dairy

---

23. Bounous G, Gold P. *The biological activity of undenatured dietary whey proteins: role of glutathione. Clin Invest Med.* 1991; 14:296-309.

cows consume alternative feed such as corn, soy and feed with added antibiotics. This diet creates a fatter cow quicker. Unlike US cattle,

New Zealand and Australian cattle consume grass that is free of herbicides and pesticides. This is a very good thing, as we should only be getting antibiotics prescribed by a doctor, not from the grocery store.

LOW GLYCEMIC INDEX IS CRITICAL

Another very important reason that these super whey protein and vegan shakes are so beneficial to us is that they have a very low glycemic index, in part because they contain prebiotic fiber which slows down the release of glucose, thus avoiding insulin spikes. In addition, prebiotic fiber multiplies and allows the body to produce more good flora (gut bacteria) critical for supporting our immune system. Any shake you consume should contain prebiotic fiber (oligosaccharides).

A shake should contain 240 calories to be classified as a meal replacement, and you want meal replacements, not a lower-calorie shake (100 to 180 calories), which is more like a snack.

GLUTATHIONE A NATURAL TOXIN HUNTER

Glutathione (found in whey protein) and selenium (a micro mineral) are critical in the fight against toxins. Glutathione is a critical substance for detoxifying the liver and every cell in the body. Its production depends on the availability of several amino acids, along with available iron and an important trace mineral called selenium. Together, these form the enzyme glutathione peroxidase, which is a step in glutathione production and metabolism.

When glutathione production is low, detoxification in the liver is seriously impaired. This means the body is less able to eliminate all toxic metals, many toxic chemicals and other substances such as biological toxins.[24]

Glutathione is needed in every cell in the body to protect cell membranes, cell proteins and DNA. It is also one of two primary ways the body detoxifies itself. Most glutathione is produced naturally in the body, but the toxins contained in most foods today diminish glutathione levels. There are supplements available containing glutathione or glutathione-sparing nutrients. However, these nutrient supplements can be difficult for the body to absorb and may only provide minor benefits. See below what Dr. Gray has to say about glutathione:

> "Every second the brain is bombarded with extra free radicals caused by nutritional deficiencies, junk food, environmental toxicity, mercury and other heavy metals, prescribed drugs, and even over-the-counter-drugs.
>
> If these extra free radicals are not stabilized by an abundance of internally produced antioxidants then oxidative stress increases. The biggest problem with these sources of extra free radicals is that they inhibit the body's ability to make the necessary glutathione. Either they deplete glutathione levels or even worse they directly stop the production of glutathione. In the case of a child with Autism, a major risk factor is the inability to make glutathione during the gestation period and after birth.

24. Wilson, 2011

A reduction in glutathione dramatically increases the child's vulnerability to oxidative stress, which derails the brain's normal development. Unable to generate enough glutathione, a fetus produces oxidative stress while in the womb. This makes the fetus more vulnerable to the extra free radicals the mother is exposed to. The biggest factors that inhibit both the mother's and the baby's ability to make glutathione are high and low blood sugar levels, fever-suppressing drugs, painkillers, and other over-the-counter-drugs, prescribed-drugs, and aluminum toxicity from antacids."

As we pointed out earlier, this undenatured whey protein has been shown to be very effective in combating oxidative stress, which is a very good thing for all of us. This again supports our goal of making you aware of what is available utilizing these preventative technologies.

INTERCONNECTIVITY IS ESSENTIAL IN TDOS SOLUTIONS

The good news is that New Zealand and Australian whey proteins are high in the amino acid cysteine, which has been shown to significantly boost glutathione levels in the body. As Dr. Gray has stated, it is always better for the body to make more glutathione on its own, instead of taking a glutathione supplement. This is a great example of the interconnectivity and the effectiveness of TDOS Solutions' combination of magnifying forces to combat the "S" –the chronic oxidative stress – in TDOS Syndrome.

Why use undenatured whey protein for fighting toxins? Many of the thousands of research studies on glutathione have revealed that an undenatured whey protein source is a great way to boost glutathione levels, which is exactly what we need to have happen. The research we have cited indicates that the ultratrace element selenium is a cofactor for cysteine, making it more effective. Cysteine plays a huge part in boosting glutathione levels. As we've discussed elsewhere, there are a wide array of minerals that make up the "Mineral Suite"; for example, some of the major minerals are, calcium, phosphorus, potassium, sodium, chloride, magnesium, and sulfur.

Some examples of micro minerals would be iron, chromium, cobalt, fluoride, and zinc. Then, there are what are referred to as ultratrace elements, including boron, bromine, and selenium, that can be added to any shake you drink.

> **NOTE:** It is always recommended to check with your health professional before embarking on any diet, exercise or nutritional regimen to determine what is best for each individual.

> **NOTE:** New Zealand or Australian undenatured whey protein and this high-grade vegan shake are very high in amino acids, which are critical food for the first brain.

MILK OR WHEY ALLERGY? THERE IS AN OPTION:

For people who are vegan or lactose intolerant, a substitute non-dairy or vegan shake can be used. There are a variety of plant-based proteins on the market. It is critical that these plant-based proteins virtually simulate the New Zealand Whey counterpart. These protein-meal supplementations should have high bioavailability, contain the critical "mineral suites" with trace micro and macro minerals. These plant-based proteins should not contain soy protein or artificial sweeteners, as they will not allow for maximizing wellness. These proteins must contain multiple plant protein sources—not a sole source. Multiple sources of plant-based proteins are necessary to simulate the effects of the whey. For example, a vegan shake just based solely on pea protein is insufficient as a sole source of protein required to do the heavy lifting in assisting the body in naturally detoxifying itself.

VEGAN SHAKES USING ONLY PEA PROTEIN

The reason a single source of vegetable protein by itself is not an effective toxin hunter is that it does not have a high enough amino acid profile to allow the body to naturally detoxify itself. To use a vegan shake with a high enough amino acid profile to be able to efficiently assist the body in the detoxification, it must contain several sources of vegetable proteins combined in one shake. When careful attention is paid to the nutritional profile, a vegan shake can be very effective in creating a preventive intervention to toxins and to living healthier longer. Whey protein is generally regarded the world over as the gold standard for amino acid profiles. The great news is that by combining several vegetable proteins, you can achieve almost the same amino acid profile as whey protein. When combined, these can provide a complete amino acid profile similar to that of a whey protein shake.

There are some additional ingredients for a world-class vegan shake. These non-dairy shakes should also contain a healthy fat source such as extra virgin olive oil powder, sunflower oil, flax, coconut oils, and MCT oils, which are critical for heart health. Also necessary are monounsaturated fats, and chia seed, omega 3, 6, and 9). And, your belly will benefit from dietary fiber that includes a mix of chia seed and gut-healthy prebiotic fiber like inulin and oligosaccharides. Additional micronutrients are also needed. You will want to make sure that the Vegan shake also contains Vitamin D-3, which works synergistically with oleic acid (from the olive oil powder) to provide great immune system support.

This vegetarian meal alternative also should possess its own "whole foods" base of micronutrients (to retain vitamins and phytochemicals) and juice powders from natural foods. These should include a variety of fruits, nuts, and vegetables, including carrots and beets.

OTHER MINERAL RECOMMENDATIONS:

SUPER MINERALS:

The following are excerpts from John Gray PhD and his amazing research:

> "While researching the work of Dr. Hans Nieper, I learned about special mineral supplements from Germany that were bonded to orotic acid, a substance high in mother's breast milk and whey protein. Unlike common mineral supplements bonded to carbonate, citrate, phosphate, ascorbate, chloride, etc., these mineral supplements from Germany were bonded to orotic acid. This allows these minerals to be freely transported across the blood-brain barrier. These mineral orotates help brain function immediately. They are super minerals for super brain

function. The brain is only 2% of your body weight but it uses 25% of your energy. Your brain needs energy and fuel to be at its peak performance. The minerals needed for optimum brain function, include iron, magnesium, zinc, and calcium, as well as trace minerals, such as chromium and selenium. If you've been having trouble concentrating, it's likely you are not getting enough of the minerals your brain needs. Research shows that magnesium can reduce irritability and hyperactivity in children with attention disorders. Iron is needed, not only to build blood cells, but is also used by the brain. Some children with iron deficiencies have demonstrated impaired intellectual performance.

These minerals include potassium, calcium, magnesium, zinc, chromium, lithium, boron and other trace minerals. All are very important to fighting the effects of poor nutrition and nutrient depletion from living in our modern world."

Activated B vitamins with sustained release technology (SRT) provides the ready-to-use, active forms needed by your body.

Every cell in the body, every second of the day and night, uses B vitamins. Running low on any one of them can create all kinds of health challenges. B vitamins help encourage mental alertness, concentration, and memory. B vitamins maintain proper functioning of the heart, nervous system and the digestive system. They support the body's ability to detoxify itself, and aid a balanced response to stress. Most B vitamin supplement products contain only the inactive forms. Inactive forms of B vitamins can be hard on the body, because they require the liver to work overtime trying to convert them so your body can absorb them. And when your body does not readily absorb them, they are quickly eliminated from the body without being used. This makes most B vitamin supplements very ineffective. Since they are water-soluble, your body cannot store them and must have a constant supply to keep body systems functioning properly. Activated B w/SRT vitamins are already converted and in the form your body can instantly use.

Activated B w/SRT B vitamins use sustained release technology for controlled absorption over eight hours. So instead of flooding the system with extra B vitamins that the body simply discards or worse, ends up using to feed unhealthy organisms, activated B w/SRT gradually releases the B vitamins in a steady stream for better use. So you get the vitamins you need, when your body needs them.

Also, when massive amounts of B vitamins are immediately released into the body, unfriendly bacteria in the digestive system may use them as a food source. This is why some people may begin to feel poorly after regular consumption of common B vitamin supplements. The sustained release technology addresses this issue by providing a steady, balanced stream of B vitamins rather than flooding the system all at once.

A recent research study confirmed that B-complex vitamins enhance mood and modulate psychological strain related to work stress. The study states that occupational stress is greater than ever in Western societies and impacts individuals and communities on many levels. In this double-blind, randomized, placebo-controlled clinical trial, 60 subjects were supplemented with a B-complex multivitamin or placebo for three months. The subjects were assessed for work demands, personality traits, mood, and work strain at the beginning of the study and again after the supplementation period.

The study showed that the subjects who received the B-complex supplement reported enhanced mood and less personal strain compared to the placebo group, even after controlling for individual differences in personality and work demands. The researchers state that this study demonstrates that 90 days of supplementation with a B-complex multivitamin modulates workplace stress. These findings may have important personal health, organizational and societal outcomes given the rising cost and incidence of workplace stress.

GRAPE SEED EXTRACT IS A POWERFUL ANTIOXIDANT THAT STRENGTHENS AND PROTECTS LIVING TISSUE

Scientific studies show that the antioxidant power of grape seed extract is 20 times more powerful than that of vitamin E and 50 times greater than that of vitamin C. Grape seed extract helps to strengthen blood vessels by increasing the tone and elasticity of capillary walls. Results from human case reports and animal studies show that grape seed extract may be useful to treat heart diseases such as high blood pressure and high cholesterol. Grape seed extract slows down the oxidation of the fats that are responsible for cholesterol. The longer it takes for fats to oxidize, the less likely they will be to clog up your veins and arteries. Grape seed may also be able to protect against Alzheimer's disease by reducing inflammation in the brain.

2009 STUDY IN NEUROTOXICITY RESEARCH

A 2009 study published in neurotoxicity research found that grape seed extract led to less inflammation of the brain. Researchers from Mount Sinai School of Medicine conducted experiments in mice with Alzheimer's disease to see if grape seeds could affect Alzheimer's disease-type cognitive deterioration. For five months, the mice received grape seed extract or water alone as a placebo treatment. The mice were then tested in various mazes to determine brain function. Brain tissue samples were also tested to see if there was evidence of Alzheimer's disease. The mice treated with grape seed extract had significantly reduced Alzheimer's disease-type cognitive deterioration as compared to the other mice.

One particular type of phenol found in grape seed is called procyanidin. It was initially discovered in 1936 by Professor Jacques Masquelier, who called it Vitamin P (although the name didn't really catch on). Procyanidins are thought to protect the body from premature aging. Procyanidins bond with collagen, the most abundant protein in the body and a key component of skin, gums, bones, teeth, hair and body tissues. The bonding promotes cell health and skin elasticity, making it seem more youthful, in a process that works almost like a natural face-lift. Procyanidins additionally help protect the body from sun damage, which can also cause premature aging of the skin.

Vitamin D is critical to the health of your brain and nervous, cardiovascular and immune systems. Many health challenges are now being linked to Vitamin D deficiency. Vitamin D is also called the sunshine vitamin because it is formed naturally in the skin with sunlight exposure. We are experiencing an unprecedented epidemic of vitamin D deficiency, resulting in more health problems, because so many people are now avoiding exposure to the sun due to the risk of skin cancer. Vitamin D supplementation is important because it's hard to get enough during long, dark, northern winters. The elderly have more difficulty synthesizing vitamin D from sunlight, and some medications interfere with vitamin D absorption and absorbing calcium, which will strengthen bones and prevent fractures.

Vitamin D plays a dual role as both a vitamin and a hormone that stimulates the body to absorb calcium. Vitamin D, calcium, and phosphorus are needed to keep bones strong. People with low vitamin D levels tend to have soft, thin bones, predisposing them to fractures, especially hip fractures. Soft bones can also cause the nagging and unremitting bone pain that many older people suffer from.

Vitamin D3 also has profound effects on the brain, including the neurotransmitters involved in depression. Both depression and suicide rates peak from January to April, when vitamin D3 levels are usually lowest. A University of Toronto study found that the incidence of depression was reduced for people taking vitamin D3 daily.

Vitamin D is produced when sunlight converts cholesterol in your skin into a form of Vitamin D3 called calciol. Then your liver hydroxylases calciol into a form called calcidiol (25-hydroxyvitamin D3). The kidneys then hydroxylate calcidiol into the active form of vitamin D called calcitriol (1,25-dihydroxy-vitamin D3). This form of vitamin D3 is derived from sheep wool lanolin. A person with fair skin with full body exposure to sunlight can produce up to 20,000 IU of vitamin D3 in just 20 minutes. Published research now suggests that people take 1,000 IU daily and up to 5,000 IU daily in winter or whenever exposure to sunlight is limited.

Omega oils are a revolutionary form of omega-3 fatty acids derived from wild salmon to support a healthy heart and brain. Omega oils boost brainpower. There's compelling evidence that the omega-3 fatty acids in fish-oil supplements can improve your mood as well as your memory and other cognitive functions. Researchers at UCLA recently discovered that people with low blood levels of omega-3 fatty acids had smaller brain volumes and performed more poorly on tests of visual memory, abstract memory and executive function than people with high levels. Danish researchers compared the diets of more than 5,000 older adults, and they found that those who ate the most fish were less likely to get dementia and more likely to maintain robust memories.

Unfortunately, many of our diets are high in omega-6 fatty acids, which are found in processed foods, red meats and cooking oils. So even if you eat a lot of fish, you still need supplements to achieve the recommended ratio of one part omega-3s to every three parts omega-6s. Vectomega contains up to 50 times higher triglyceride fish oil than other omega oil supplements because Vectomega is not fish oil. The fatty acids in wild salmon are bound to phospholipids instead of triglycerides, making them more stable. Vectomega is produced with enzymes and cold water, using no heat, pressure or solvents. Vectomega does not cause gastric upset or the "fish burps" common to the use of commercial fish oils.

NOTE: The authors of this book receive no compensation from referring readers to John Gray's Mars Venus website, where many of these vitamins and minerals can be purchased.

MORE SUPER FOODS FOR YOUR FIRST BRAIN

Below, you will find suggestions for super foods and supplements that work with and assist the first brain to work at optimal levels. The foods and mineral supplements recommended in this section will literally provide that extra mental boost we are all looking for. The trace mineral deficiency in humans is a major missing piece of the puzzle when looking at supplying the body with the proper foods, supplements and minerals. Trace minerals provide the basic foundation by allowing increased absorption of food and supplements into the body on a cellular level. John Gray's suggestions for specific foods, minerals and supplements come from 15 years of his own personal research with thousands of participants at his wellness seminars.

Due to Dr. Gray's own trials and tribulations, he took it upon himself to find what works and what doesn't and ultimately put together a comprehensive list of the best of the best. He was also a pioneer in finding ways to maximize what he was putting in his body by making sure the body was open and accepting of these powerful brain foods. By adding certain ingredients, the body literally opens up and becomes like a sponge, capable of absorbing the best each food, vitamin and mineral has to offer.

The first brain needs specific foods to maximize its potential. If you are going to feed yourself, it seems logical to assume that the first thing you would want to feed is your first brain. There has been a lot of research done on the best possible foods and/or regimes for the first brain. The following is a list of additional foods that have been shown to support our first brain.

ESSENTIAL FATTY ACIDS. These are not made in the human body, and instead have to be obtained from outside sources (food). They are therefore critical for maximizing the potential of our first brain.

The following is a list of some of the best-known sources of essential fatty acids:

- Salmon
- Trout
- Mackerel
- Herring
- Sardines
- COD

(Fish provide a natural source of Essential Fatty Acids).

ADDITIONAL SOURCES OF ESSENTIAL FATTY ACIDS:
- Flax Seed Oil
- Walnut Oil
- Olive Oil

- Pumpkin seeds are high in zinc, which has been shown to be essential for brain function, including supporting better memory.

In a study, it was revealed that vitamin E also supports many healthy brain functions.

GREAT SOURCES OF VITAMIN E:

- Walnuts: Walnuts are rich in vitamin E, an antioxidant that researchers from Chicago Rush University Medical Center have associated with a lower risk of developing Alzheimer's disease.[25]

- Eggs: eggs contain high amounts of choline. A study at Boston University said that consumption of choline had positive results with memory.[26]

- Brown rice

- Pumpkin seeds

- Olives

- Asparagus

- Leafy green vegetables

- Tomatoes: Dr. Gray pointed out that the reduction of free radicals due to oxidative stress is very important for optimum brain function. Lycopene found in tomatoes is very high in antioxidants, which are very effective against free radicals. This is good for the brain and for the rest of the

---

25. Source Alzheimer's Research Center

26. For more info: http://www.rd.com/slideshows/best-brain-food/#ixzz3PlijxGoD

body as well. Adding more tomatoes to your diet is an easy and effective way to boost the antioxidant capability in your body, and your brain will thank you![27]

- Broccoli: Vitamin K found in broccoli supports brain power.

- Avocados: Avocados are almost as good as blueberries at promoting brain health.[28]

- Blueberries: At Tufts University, they have shown that the consumption of blueberries can support short-term memory. This seems like a simple and wonderful addition to any sensible nutritional regime.

- Kale: Kale has also been shown to be very beneficial in supporting brain health because of its extremely high antioxidant make up.[29]

- Spinach: Spinach has very high antioxidant properties because of its high content of lutein. Spinach is not just for Popeye's muscles.

PLEASE NOTE that there are certainly more foods and supplements for the first brain than the ones listed here.

In particular, as we pointed out in *Mars Venus Super Minerals*, minerals for men and women contain high amounts of the nutrients that have been shown to support the production of healthy brain chemicals thanks to the work of Dr. John Gray.

27. Source: American Journal of Epidemiology

28. For more info, read http://www.rd.com/slideshows/best-brain-food/#ixzz3PliWUbEe

29. http://www.rd.com/slideshows/best-brain-food/#ixzz3PIj8IkG3

PURIFIED OR FILTERED WATER:

Water is a critical element for brain health. According to Feredoon Batamanghelidj, MD, the human brain is approximately 70% water. If you are not consuming enough water every day, the dehydration process starts immediately and is detrimentally bad for the brain. We have seen, in the movies, men at sea forced to drink seawater and within a few short hours, they become deranged and delusional, and ultimately die from lack of pure fresh water for their brains. It is suggested as a simple rule of thumb, in order to just maintain a baseline hydration in the body; every person should consume half of their body weight in ounces of water every day. This rule does not take in any daily variables such as consuming sodas, coffee, alcohol, etc. If these beverages are part of your day to day, you need to con-sume more water than the suggested rule of half your bodyweight in ounces.

GO NUTS:

A study published in the, "American Journal of Epidemiology", suggests that a good intake of vitamin E might help to prevent cog-nitive decline, particularly in the elderly. Nuts are a great source of vitamin E, along with leafy green vegetables, asparagus, olives, seeds, eggs, brown rice and whole grains.

BRAIN POWER SUPPLEMENTS:

Although research linking diet and dementia is still in its infancy, there are a few important relationships between nutrients and brain health that are worth exploring. Having a nourishing, well-rounded diet gives the brain the best chance of avoiding disease. If your diet is unbalanced for whatever reason, you may want to consider a multivitamin and mineral complex and an omega-3 fatty acid supplement to help supplement a few of the essentials. If you are considering taking a supplement, it is best to discuss this with a doctor or qualified healthcare professional.

All health content on bbcgoodfood.com is provided for general information only, and should not be treated as a substitute for the medical advice of your own doctor or any other health care professional. If you have any concerns about your general health, you should contact your local health care provider. See their website's terms and conditions for more information.

7

Food for the 2ⁿᵈ Brain

Science now believes that our second brain is the primary driving force behind our thoughts, feeling, and emotions, and to a large degree, who we are.

Dr. Ruggiero conveys the importance of what we feed the second brain really can make a huge impact on how we feel and act in our everyday lives.

The foods we consume can have a profound impact on our happiness, our optimism, and our zest for life.

Before revealing the best foods for the second brain, it is important that Dr. Ruggiero explains how critically important food really is to all three brains. Food is not only a source of nourishment but, more importantly, it is the carrier of genetic information that is the operating and communication system to enable your three brains to work together.

The microbiome relies on a robust and healthy second brain (our gut bacteria and immune system) in order for it to be an effective operating system for the human body. The old saying "food matters" has far-reaching implications. If you want to maximize your quality of life, what you put in your mouth is not just for your stomach. It is also for the other 99%.

BEHAVIOR IS DICTATED BY WHAT WE EAT

So essentially, this puts us in a very awkward position, because our behavior is dictated by what we eat—not only due to the proteins and the fat and the calories, but also because what we eat we contributes to the flora in our gut. This flora is what drives us to behave in one way or another. So it's a complete revolutionary thought that I myself still have difficulty grasping, but I'm so excited to be now in this age where we're making such important discoveries, and learning that maybe—maybe—we can even influence these things.

MICROBIAL STRAINS MAY HOLD THE KEY TO WHO WE ARE

Just imagine that I discover which microbial strains give us courage, so to speak, or a sense of honesty (which is desperately needed in these days), and I can put those strains into a yogurt and drink them and become courageous and honest, which is a rare combination. Can you imagine how I could positively influence my behavior without the necessity of taking psychoactive drugs or any types of drugs, or knocking my head on the wall? It's a very interesting revolution; a new way of thinking.

YOU ARE WHAT YOU EAT

We often hear the saying "You are what you eat" referenced as a joke. But it's *not* a joke. You are more materially what you eat than you might believe.

Today we can go beyond this narrow concept of eating as a source of proteins, sugars, fats, calories, minerals, and so on. What we eat essentially is genetic information that we communicate to our genes. Then, the genes interpret this genetic information and give commands to our cells. If this genetic information is corrupted or incomplete (depleted) due to eating nutritionally deficient foods, our quality of life suffers.

GENES COMMUNICATE WHAT THEY RECEIVE FROM FOOD

Our genes are set up to communicate whatever genetic information they receive from food, be it pristine or corrupted genetic intelligence, to our cells. If food is delivering inadequate, incomplete or corrupted information, the genes will simply carry out their job and pass on this bad information. Our cells can only deal with this information when they receive it and react accordingly.

It is pretty apparent that the more corrupted genetic information communicated to our cells, the greater the likelihood that the cells will become corrupted and begin to mutate. That is not the formula for maximizing our quality-of-life potential, our wellness potential or our ability to live healthier longer.

WE EAT GENETIC INFORMATION

You know, one of the gourmet things in Switzerland is cheese—a fermented milk product. Every time I eat some good gruyere cheese or some Hamiter cheese, I'm actually eating genetic information. This is because all the bacteria that have brought about the fermentation process of this delicious cheese have produced proteins, nucleic acids—information. So I'm not simply eating something nutritious or something fat, something good or bad for my cholesterol. I'm eating precious genetic information. So I am what I eat, not only because of the proteins and the fat, but because of the genetic information that the food is contributing to my body.

INTERCONNECTIVITY OF ALL THREE BRAINS

Here, I continue my conversation with Dr. Ruggiero.

PETER: Dr. Ruggiero, let me see if I've got this correct. The food we supply to the second brain (our gut microbes, bacteria and neurons of the gut) creates genetic information that is communicated and used by all three of our brains.

In essence the microbiome (the third brain) communicates directly to the second brain, which in turn sends genetic information through our genes to the first brain. Is it then the third brain that has the ability, through its dopamine receptors, to actually go directly to the first brain?

NOTE: Dr. Ruggiero already explained in great detail how the microbiome is able to communicate, or in essence, talk to the other two brains in a common language used by our DNA.

DR. RUGGIERO: "Yes. As a matter of fact, today, for example, we are treating a psychiatric illness by working on the third brain. We will be able in the very near future (more research is needed), if not right now, to greatly improve psychiatric challenges by simply giving somebody this super yogurt we discovered.

PETER: I think we can see how critically important feeding our second brain the proper foods can be for our quality of life.

DR. RUGGIERO: In our more than three decades of research, working directly with patients on their nutritional intake as the cornerstone to maintaining wellness, we have discovered what we believe is the single most important food for the second brain.

For some time now, we have used, with great success, an undenatured whey protein specifically from New Zealand with our healthy patients as well as patients we were treating for many serious health challenges.

In the last year we have discovered an enhanced New Zealand whey protein that has, in our opinion, magnified the benefits we have already seen over many years from using a traditional New Zealand whey protein. Our patients and individuals on this regimen have been thriving and truly experiencing increased wellness.

PETER: For consumers, putting together this formulation for the New Zealand whey, combined with the complex added nutrients, amino acid profile, prebiotic fibers and trace-minerals, may be extremely costly and time consuming. For those who choose to get started with this protocol as directed by Dr. Ruggiero and his team, we have found a convenient and affordable way to offer this formulation to you. For more information, please contact us at www.yourthirdbrain.com. For the kitchen chemists, we have a recipe for you to follow. To formulate food for the first and second brains, we would like to share with you what you will want to add to what we believe is already the best protein source in the world. As we mentioned throughout this book, the best food in the world for all of us is mothers' breast milk. By way of review, or in case it was unclear, mothers' breast milk is comprised of approximately 60% whey protein and 40% milk protein. By contrast, much of the milk we have available to us in North America is only 20% whey and 80% milk protein.

Due to the important ratios of milk proteins in mother's breast milk, we have found the New Zealand whey protein more appealing, as it is comprised of 60% whey and 40% milk protein. We consume this ourselves and have strongly recommended it as a foundation to supporting quality of life

Utilizing this New Zealand Whey Protein, we have created a "Super Shake".

The Super Shake Meal Specifics:

- Use an undenatured New Zealand whey protein processed using low-temperature, high-filtration pasteurization, as opposed to the high-heat pasteurization typically used in North America, which greatly reduces the amino acids available to the human body.

- Include prebiotic fiber – approximately 6-9 grams based upon 24-36 g of the protein – which should primarily be from flaxseed and isomaltooligosaccharides. Not all fiber is the same, and this prebiotic fiber in particular is so important to our bodies because it feeds healthy flora (good bacteria) in our digestive tract. It also is an important factor in regulating the release of Glucose and providing a very low glycemic index. This is beneficial to our overall health and quality of life.

- No artificial flavorings.
- No artificial sweeteners. Use a pure and organic stevia as the sweetener (stevia contains no sugar and is naturally derived from the stevia plant). As a result, these shakes taste great, yet they have a very low glycemic index. Add good fats, including olive oil, sunflower oil, and coconut oil.
- No soy or soy-derived ingredients.
- The super shake should also contain the enzyme Lactase. Although these New Zealand Shakes contain almost zero lactose, the addition of the lactase will further reduce any lactose present. Thus, many people who are lactose intolerant are able to easily digest these shakes with this added enzyme.
- Add multiple proteases, enzymes that help to break down protein into particles called peptides that make the protein much easier to absorb. These are the proteases you want to add: (from Aspergillus oryzae), bromelain (from Ananas comosus), papain (from Carica papaya), acid stable protease (from Aspergillus niger).

- In addition, the super shake contains up to 70 major minerals, minor minerals (called trace minerals) and Ultratrace elements. These minerals have been called the spark plugs of life. These minerals are the co-factors for enzyme reactions, which play a crucial role in the most efficient functioning of our enzymes.

- The super shake must also include vitamin D-3 and oleic acid (from olive oil). You will learn about their critical importance in magnifying the impact of The Microbiome Protocol, the food for Your Third Brain.

> **NOTE:** All of these, the proteases, minerals, lactose, pre-biotic fiber, and vitamin D-3 and oleic acid, are included in this new Super Shake. Thus they significantly enhance and improve the Super Shake we now use with all of our patients.

- No gluten (absent in New Zealand whey).

OUR SUPER FOOD DISCOVERY

The other critical component to our overall quality-of-life approach is this super food we created with a proprietary combination of milk, colostrum, and 40 strains of bacteria in a fermentation process that we have discovered and created after many, many scientific experiments.

> "Let me say again as we have stated over and over in this book. We always use the nutritional intelligence we have gained in conjunction with and never as a substitute for conventional medical treatments, drugs, therapies, approaches or protocols.

It has been our observation with our patients as well as ourselves that no therapy or medical intervention can overcome a poor diet. That is our fundamental guiding principle that we continue to use today.

It is always recommended that you do check with your doctor and or health professional before embarking on any nutritional plan. As no one nutritional technology or product is the answer. It is also important again to state that none of these statements have been approved by the FDA.

We will say however that there are now many observational studies that show very promising and encouraging results and to give us hope for the best quality of life."

OTHER SUPER FOODS FOR THE SECOND BRAIN

Use organic when possible

- Asparagus
- Garlic
- Tomatoes
- Onions
- Carrots
- Radishes
- Probiotics
- Prebiotic fiber from nature
- You may also want to use:

- Sauerkraut
- Vegetables

Other ingredients that are very good as part of your nutrition are:
- Turmeric
- Cinnamon
- Grape seed extract—also mentioned as food for the first brain

As more and more research emerges, there may be a whole new host of nutritional approaches to magnify and enhance the health of the second brain.

We also mentioned the importance in our chapter on the second brain that toxins, nutritional deficiency, overweightness and stress also can work to destroy the good bacteria in the gut. Remember, it is critically important to carefully follow your doctor's instructions when consuming antibiotics, as the misuse or overuse of antibiotics has drastically negative effects on the second and third brains.

8

Food for the Third Brain: A New Super Food

Dr. Ruggiero's discovery of this food for the third brain sits at the pinnacle of his career of medical and scientific breakthroughs. He and his colleagues are on the cutting edge of changing how we view maximizing our wellness potential by supporting the immune system and its amazing job of keeping us healthy. This is the story of a career of research, experimentation and discovering the *dessert cup*, as Dr. Ruggiero affectionately refers to this nutritional discovery, as told by the doctor himself.

Since 2009, my research group at the University of Firenze involved working in the field of immunotherapy. Immunotherapy is an approach that has been recently rediscovered and consists of empowering the immune system so that it can attack cells infected by viruses or other pathogens, including cancer cells as well as cells that have undergone degeneration. The main difference with the classical pharmacological therapy is in the target; most drugs try to kill the cancer cells, or the pathogenic microbes. In an immunotherapeutic approach, the target is the immune system or particular cells of the immune system like macrophages, with the objective of "arming" them so that they can go and kill the cancer cells or those infected by microbes in the most natural way. We will cover more on immunotherapy in the next chapter, but this approach to strengthening the immune system set the tone for the discovery of food for the third brain, which I call the dessert cup.

Macrophages, which have already been described elsewhere in this book, are the natural killers, lymphocytes, often abbreviated as NK cells. They are a type of cytotoxic lymphocytes critical to the innate immune system. Here, innate means a part of the immune system that works independently of the threats that we encounter. In other words, they're a part of the immune system that's always ready to work, even if it has never encountered a given menace before.

NK cells provide rapid responses to viral-infected cells and respond to tumor formation; they are very fast, with a reaction time of around three days. NK cells are unique among the other cells of the immune system, since they are the first to recognize stressed cells, thus allowing for a much faster immune reaction. They were designated "natural killers" because of the initial notion that they do not require previous activation to kill cells that are somehow dangerous for the organism. In addition to this fundamental role in the innate immune response, NK cells also play important roles in the adaptive immune responses, and because of this, they are considered very promising candidates for potential immunotherapies of cancer, viral infections and neurodegenerative diseases.

CAN NK AND MACROPHAGES BE STIMULATED?

Thus, our research focused on the way to stimulate macrophages and NK cells, and in addition to this goal, we wanted to find a natural way to perform this task. The search for a natural way derived from the rather obvious observation that you cannot take synthetic drugs for a long time without side effects. Conversely, if we could find a way to stimulate macrophages and NK cells in a natural way, possibly through nutrition, this approach could have been adopted for life, with obvious benefits not only for the prevention of diseases, but also for the increase in general wellness and fitness and to help support graceful aging.

We knew that there were two completely natural things that, at the same time, stimulated macrophages and NK cells:

1. Vitamin D.

2. Fermented milk products such as yogurts and kefirs. Currently, there are more than 1,700 peer-reviewed papers in PubMed that deal with, "vitamin D and macrophages" and 88 papers on "vitamin D and NK cells". The total number of papers on "vitamin D and the immune system" is around 3,200; this is truly a huge number testifying to the interest of the international scientific community in this topic. Also, the topic of fermented milk products and the immune system is a hot one, and a search for "probiotics and immune system" yields more than 1,600 papers.

20 YEARS OF EXPERIENCE WITH VITAMIN D AXIS

We were in the lucky position of having some 20 years of experience in the so-called vitamin D axis. We were considered world experts in this field, and we have published 21 peer-reviewed papers on this topic, including an invited review for the very prestigious journal, "Kidney International."[30] Vitamin D, being synthesized in the kidney, plays a crucial role in chronic kidney disease, and we were asked by the Editors of the Journal to write a commentary on the most adequate dosage of vitamin D in these pathologies.

We were also well positioned in the field of fermented milk products and the immune system, and in 2011, we were invited to present our work on this topic at the 6th Conference of International AIDS Society Conference in Rome, on HIV pathogenesis, treatment and prevention. A study of ours (abstract CDB 269) describing, among other things, the role of fermented milk products in stimulating the immune system, was presented and placed on the CD-ROM given to the thousands of participants from all over the world.

Thus, we had the expertise to engineer a food that could exploit the competence that we had accumulated in more than 30 years of research. As a matter of fact, the first paper that I published when I had just graduated from the Medical School of the University of Firenze was on the role of food (contaminated with a fungus) in the development of liver cancer in sub-Saharan African populations.[31]

---

30. Chronic kidney disease and vitamin D: how much is adequate? Ruggiero M, Pacini S. Kidney Int. 2009 Nov;76(9):931-3.

31. This paper (Ruggiero, M. and Nicastro, C.: Il problema delle micotossine nei paesi tropicali. J. Agricult. Environ. for Intl. Dev. 74: 221-235, 1980) is listed in the National Agricultural Library of the United States Department of Agriculture under the keywords: "feeds; foods; tropic".

30 YEARS TO DEVELOP SUPER FERMENTED MILK

With this scientific knowledge, we decided to develop the best-fermented milk product that had ever been engineered, taking inspiration from the almost miraculous work of nature. We were interested, in particular, in those strains of microbes that are associated with longevity and health. In fact, it is well assessed that consumption of fermented milk products is associated with longevity. For example, in the year 2000, a group of researchers studied 162 self-sufficient residents in a public home for the elderly in Rome, Italy, to evaluate the association between the consumption of specific food groups and nutrients and overall five-year survival, and they demonstrated that "frequent consumption of citrus fruit, milk, and yogurt, low consumption of meat, and high intake of vitamin C, riboflavin, and linoleic acid are associated with longevity."[32] In another study conducted in Warsaw, it was observed that centenarians ate yogurt more often.[33]

32. Epidemiology. 2000 Jul;11(4):440-5. Diet and overall survival in a cohort of very elderly people. Fortes C, Forastiere F, Farchi S, Rapiti E, Pastori G, Perucci CA.

33. Rocz Panstw Zakl Hig. 2007;58(1):279-86. The nutritional habits among centenarians living in Warsaw. Kołłajtis-Dołowy A, Pietruszka B, Kałuza J, Pawlińiska-Chmara R, Broczek K, Mossakowska M.

LONGEVITY CAN BE ENHANCED BY MANIPULATING GASTROINTESTINAL MICROBES

These recent studies indexed in PubMed reverberate the century old hypothesis of Nobel Laureate Ilya Ilyich Mechnikov who, by the way, was the first to discover and describe the macrophages. Mechnikov hypothesized that longevity could be enhanced by manipulating gastrointestinal microbes using naturally fermented foods. In fact, he developed a theory that aging is caused by toxic bacteria in the gut and that lactic acid could prolong life. Based on this theory, he drank sour milk every day. He wrote three books on this subject: *Immunity in Infectious Diseases*, *The Nature of Man*, and *The Prolongation of Life: Optimistic Studies*. This latter book, together with Metchnikoff's studies into the potential life-lengthening properties of lactic acid bacteria (*Lactobacillus Delbrueckii subspecie Bulgaricus*), inspired Japanese scientist Minoru Shirota to begin investigating a causal relationship between bacteria and good intestinal health, which eventually led to the worldwide marketing of kefir and other fermented milk drinks and probiotics. This legacy is so strong that it is still quoted in articles published in January 2015 such as the one entitled "Human milk: Mother Nature's prototypical probiotic food?"[34]

THE FIVE HUGE CHALLENGES TO OVERCOME

But, of course, being in the first century of the third millennium AD, we could not simply rediscover yogurt or kefir. We were facing five different challenges:

---

34. Adv Nutr. 2015 Jan 15;6(1):112-23. McGuire MK, McGuire MA.

1. Identify the molecules produced by the microbes that were responsible for the well-known neuroprotective support, supporting the immune system, and supporting the graceful aging of fermented milk products.

2. Identify the microbes responsible for the production of these molecules.

3. Assess the role of the different components of the vitamin D axis in this context.

4. Create a unique array of microbes and molecules that could reproduce, as a food, the healthy core human microbiome.

5. Make all this so simple that it could be performed in a common home kitchen.

We immediately realized that we could not count solely on our abilities as cellular and molecular biologists; we needed a deeper insight into the complexity of the interconnections between the genetic information that were at work. And, in order to do so, we needed the help of a technique that had never been applied before to cellular or molecular biology: the deconstruction.

The French philosopher Jacques Derrida described this technique, and it is considered one of the most obscure and difficult to master concepts in modern philosophy, possibly even more obscure than Goedel's theorems of incompleteness. According to Wikipedia, the word deconstruction means:

"In the 1980s designated more loosely a range of theoretical enterprises in diverse areas of the humanities and social sciences including—in addition to philosophy and literature—law, anthropology, historiography, linguistics, sociolinguistics, psychoanalysis, political theory, feminism, and gay and lesbian studies. Deconstruction still has a major influence in the academe of Continental Europe, South America and everywhere Continental philosophy is predominant, particularly in debates around ontology, epistemology, ethics, aesthetics, hermeneutics, and the philosophy of language. It also influenced architecture (in the form of deconstructivism), music, art, and art criticism."

THE TECHNIQUE DEVELOPED FOR THIS SUPER FOOD HAD NEVER BEEN APPLIED TO CELLULAR OR MOLECULAR BIOLOGY.

However, until our approach, this technique has never been applied to cellular and molecular biology. One may wonder, therefore, what a philosophical enterprise has to do with cells and genes, or, even worse, with yogurts and kefirs, except for the fact that maybe philosophers too enjoy yogurts.

However, if we further explore the essence of deconstruction, following the divulging words of Wikipedia, we learn that:

"Deconstruction denotes the pursuing of the meaning of a text to the point of exposing the supposed contradictions and internal oppositions upon which it is founded—supposedly showing that those foundations are irreducibly complex, unstable, or impossible. It is an approach that may be deployed in philosophy, in literary analysis, and even in the analysis of scientific writings. Deconstruction generally tries to demonstrate that any text is not a discrete whole but contains several irreconcilable and contradictory meanings; that any text therefore has more than one interpretation; that the text itself links these interpretations inextricably; that the incompatibility of these interpretations is irreducible; and thus that an interpretative reading cannot go beyond a certain point. Derrida refers to this point as an "aporia" in the text; thus, deconstructive reading is termed "aporetic." He insists that meaning is made possible by the relations of a word to other words within the network of structures that language is."

LIFE IS GENETIC INFORMATION CONTAINED IN OUR DNA

In essence, our reasoning was the following: life is genetic information contained in DNA. This genetic information is in the form of letters (the bases of DNA) that form words, (the genes) that can be read. Therefore, the genetic information in a genome is a text that needs to be interpreted. In our body, there are many texts under the form of different genomes, the human genome and the microbial genomes. The microbial genes outnumber the human genes 100 to 1.

Milk itself, and fermented milk products even more, are ensembles of microbes, *i.e.* genomes, *i.e.* texts that need to be interpreted. If we can interpret (deconstruct) those texts, then we can succeed in reconstructing the original text that is our ultimate goal, the uncorrupted, primeval, healthy human core microbiome.

GENETIC INFORMATION IN THE HUMAN BODY AND FERMENTED MILK HAD TO BE INTERPRETED AS TEXT

In other words, we reasoned that we had to interpret the genetic information in the human body and in a fermented milk product as if they were two texts, each one composed by a number of other texts. To give an example, it is as if we were to compare the information in a hard copy of the Encyclopedia Britannica (a text composed of several texts) with the information in the website of Wikipedia. Although the information came from different media and is organized differently, each source still hopefully contains a common core of knowledge.

GENETIC INFORMATION IS CONTAINED IN SEQUENCES OF OUR DNA LIKE IN THE ENGLISH LANGUAGE

The comparison with the analysis of the texts in Wikipedia is all the more apt to understand the enormity of our task. I think that I am reading words in Wikipedia and I have to understand the meaning of the text composed by those words; in reality, there are no words, but strings of 0 and 1 in the binary code that are transformed into words by the computer program. Therefore, there is a fundamental language with its rules (the binary code), and in Wittgenstein's style, a superimposed language (the words in English) that has to be consistent with the binary code. In our case, there is the genetic information contained in the sequence of bases in DNA that is equivalent to the binary code. And, superimposed to this fundamental language, there is the information in the sequence of amino acids forming the proteins that make the cells, and this is the equivalent of the words in a natural language like English.

WE HAD TWO ENORMOUS TEXTS TO COMPARE TO UNDERSTAND IN DNA AND PROTEINS

In other words, not only did we have two enormous texts to compare and understand, but we also had to work at two different levels, the level of the genetic information contained in all the DNAs and the level of the functional information contained in the proteins.

The description of the methods that we used to apply the deconstruction to this humongous task may be too complex to be described and, therefore, I am giving just a few examples of what we did by following the teaching of Derrida.

FOOD IS INFORMATION THAT HAD TO BE ENGINEERED FOR THE HUMAN MICROBIOME

Il n'y a pas de hors-texte (there is no outside-text). All the information that we had to study and interpret was in the DNA and in the proteins. Food is information, and this was the information that we had to study, deconstruct and possibly reconstruct if we wanted to engineer a food that is the human microbiome.

Any text is not a discrete whole but contains several irreconcilable and contradictory meanings; any text therefore has more than one interpretation. We had to find these contradictions and interpret them. For example, the same microorganism may be beneficial or pathogenic, depending on the context. Or, the same protein can perform opposite functions (stimulate and inhibit), or different proteins can perform the same function (*e.g.* stimulate).

The text itself links these interpretations inextricably; the incompatibility of these interpretations is irreducible; thus, an interpretative reading cannot go beyond a certain point. We had to understand that we could not go beyond a certain point in the interpretation of the multitude of texts that were confronting us. And this statement of Derrida was not so different, in essential principle, from the theorems of incompleteness of Goedel. Therefore, we had to arrive at the deepest level of interpretation and stop there if we wished to reconstruct information that made sense, i.e. the uncorrupted human microbiome.

In fact, *meaning is made possible by the relations of a word to other words within the network of structures that language is.* That is; only if we understood the relations between the words in the different texts, (the genes and the proteins of the microbes and of the human) can we reach the concept of a meaning. And only with this concept can we recreate the same concept in a super food.

YEARS OF SLEEPLESS NIGHTS TO SOLVE THE PUZZLE

It took years of sleepless nights in front of the computer before I could find the solution to such an enormous task of interpretation, but eventually I succeeded. There was no "Eureka" moment here, but rather a slow increase in the awareness of the meaning of this miraculous assembly that is the human with its microbiome was progressively revealed.

THE FOOD FOR THE THIRD BRAIN IS CREATED... IN MY KITCHEN

At that point, once the realization was perfected, the rest was kitchen work. Mix the microbial strains according to the intrinsic meaning of their genetic information and their relation with the human information; give them the appropriate environment and food, *et voilà* (as Derrida would have exclaimed). In a cup, you have the core microbiome, the third brain, the immune system, the cardiovascular support, all you need for the development and function of your other brains. And the taste is not bad!

My comments about Dr. Ruggiero and his work:

"Dr. Ruggiero is a very humble genius, and I so respect this about him. We are so privileged to have such an amazing pioneer to bring us to the discovery of the dessert cup, as he calls it, for humankind. Not just to enjoy, but also to embrace in such a way that it may in fact greatly increase the quality of our lives for decades.

It is important to emphasize again and again that food for the third brain does not replace our brilliant medical interventions, strategies, drugs or protocols. Rather, it's a natural tool to help support our quality of life at the highest possible levels. Dr. Ruggiero and his colleagues are continuing their tireless research in molecular biology and nutritional science to create even better and more powerful nutritional support for this natural world and universe of the microbiome.

9

The Microbiome Protocol
and Regimen

INTRODUCTION – THE MICROBIOME PROTOCOL

The Microbiome Protocol is based on more than 30 years of scientific research in the fields of molecular biology, neuroscience, and oncology. The aim of the Microbiome Protocol is to support the immune system, cardiovascular health, neuron health, and graceful aging. The purpose of the protocol is to reconstitute the genetic information for the healthy core microbiome.

The Microbiome Protocol was developed as a general protocol and maintenance program to support optimal health and youthful aging. The protocol was developed based on the new discoveries of the microbiome as well as the principles of the Allgemeine Pathologie (German for general pathology). This discipline focuses on the common characteristics shared by different diseases. In fact, although diseases have different causes (aetiology) and different ways to progress (pathogenesis), they share core features at the cellular and molecular levels.

The Microbiome Protocol is based on three tenets:

1. Supporting nutrition that helps the microbiome (The Microbiome Protocol Regimen)
2. Supporting the immune system
3. Supporting the reconstitution of the microbiome

The Microbiome Protocol is not a replacement for conventional or western medicine treatments or protocols. It was developed to work in conjunction with other health care regimens. Thus, the Microbiome Protocol can be implemented in conjunction with any other type of therapeutic approach, whether conventional or complementary.

DISCLAIMER: The Microbiome Protocol and Microbiome Protocol Regimen are not intended to cure, treat, diagnose, or make any medical claims whatsoever. The statements contained in this document have not been evaluated by the FDA. It is always recommended to consult with a medical professional or health professional before embarking on any new nutritional or dietary approach.

THE MICROBIOME: AN ORGAN THAT HAS BEEN IGNORED FOR MILLENNIA

The National Institute of Health (NIH) has invested over 150 million dollars on the Human Microbiome Project.

According to NIH:

> "The typical healthy person is inhabited with trillions of microbes. To better understand the role of these organisms across our body sites, we must catalogue and analyze the organisms, and see how they interact with our cells. A new analysis of healthy microbiomes has found that each person's microbiome is unique. Therefore, two healthy people may have very different microbial communities but still be healthy. Strikingly, the researchers found that although unique, certain communities could be used to predict characteristics. For example, whether you were breastfed as an infant and even your level of education could be predicted based on microbial communities across varying body sites.[35]

> Research has shown that microbial communities from varying body sites on the same individual were predictive for others. For example, gut communities could be predicted by examining the oral community, even though these communities are vastly different from each other.

---

35. Penders et al. (2006)

Taken together, this new analysis will help pave the
way for future studies that can begin to use microbial
communities as a basis for personalizing therapies and
possibly to assess the risk for certain diseases."[36]

The concept of the microbiome emerged shortly after the characterization of the human genome. As a matter of fact, the suffix "ome" derives from the information that we gathered from studying the human genome. The current definition of the human genome, as we can find it in Wikipedia, is: *"The human genome is the complete set of genetic information for humans (Homo sapiens sapiens). This information is encoded as DNA sequences within the 23 chromosome in cell nuclei and in a small DNA molecule found within individual mitochondria".* According to this definition, the genetic information for a human is encoded in about 22,000 genes that are responsible for the synthesis and functions of all proteins, cells, and ultimately our organs.

The human microbiome being developed by the National Institute of Health demonstrated that the total number of microbial cells found in association with humans might exceed the total number of cells making up the human body by a factor of ten-to-one.

The total number of genes associated with the human microbiome could exceed the total number of human genes by more than a factor of 360-to-1. Organisms thought to be found in the human microbiome, however, can generally be categorized as bacteria (the majority), members of domain Archaea, yeasts, and single-celled eukaryotes, as well as various helminth parasites and viruses, the

---

36. http://commonfund.nih.gov/hmp/programhighlights#biome

latter including viruses that infect the cellular microbiome organisms (e.g., bacteriophages, the viruses of bacteria).

The weight of this organ is about 2 Kg (approximately 4.5 pounds) and it plays a fundamental role in the development of all other organs as well as in their function throughout all phases of human life, from birth to old age.

Referencing the University of Utah again:

> "As researchers learn more about the microbes that keep us healthy, we are coming to understand how subtle imbalances in our microbial populations can also cause disease—and how restoring the balance may lead to cures. Our new understanding may lead to more focused and effective treatments. Unlike modern antibiotics, which kill good microbes along with the bad, new drugs may kill only harmful bacteria while leaving the friendly ones alone. Others may nurture friendly bacteria, helping them out compete the harmful ones."[37]

The goal of the Microbiome Protocol and the Microbiome Protocol Regimen is fully consistent with the above statements and it is precisely intended to:

1. Restore the balance of the microbiome that may lead to an improvement of health and our quality of life.

---

37. From The University of Utah Health Sciences Department. This work was supported by an award from the National Institute of Allergy and Infectious Diseases (NIAID), one of the National Institutes of Health. Grant number R25AI095212. 2011

2. Nurture friendly bacteria, helping them outcompete the harmful ones.

3. To provide adequate nutrition to the supporting systems of the microbiome.

The human microbiome needs appropriate nutrition in order to maintain its properties, and a healthy microbiome is essential for proper nutrient absorption. This proper nutrition is what makes up The Microbiome Protocol Regimen.

According to the University of Utah:

> "The Food and Agriculture Organization of the United Nations estimates that nearly a billion people around the world either don't have enough to eat or are missing important vitamins and minerals. In children, malnutrition can lead to lifelong health problems.
>
> Malnutrition isn't simply a matter of lacking calories and nutrients. Some people eat enough nutrients but can't absorb them. One clue about the role of microbes came from looking at identical twins, one twin undernourished and the other one not. The twins had the same genes, and they ate the same food—but they had different gut microbiota.
>
> Our microbial communities are established during our first few years, and they influence our health for life. If we learn more about the relationship between microbes and nutrition, we may be able to help babies grow healthy microbes right from the start. By manipulating the

microbiome, doctors may be able to help patients take in more nutrients from essentially the same food."

In order to maintain a healthy microbiome, it is critical that it be fed a diet that is rich in proteins and low in refined carbohydrates (simple sugars).

It is well known that a high-protein/low-carbohydrate (simple sugars) regimen is essential in almost all chronic conditions. For example, when dealing with the complementary treatments of severe health challenges, the Microbiome Protocol is consistent with the 90-year-old observation of Professor Otto Warburg, who demonstrated how cancer cells are dependent on glycolysis.

Consistent with this approach, our research group has been working, for about 30 years, on the role of glycolysis in carcinogenesis and other human diseases, and it has published 13 papers on the role of byproducts of glycolysis (diacylglycerol) in cancer as well as in neurodegenerative diseases, chronic kidney disease and cardiovascular disease.[38]

---

38. For review on these papers on glucose metabolism and human diseases, and peer-reviewed papers that are indexed in PubMed, please see additional studies in the Appendix.

INTRODUCTION TO THE MICROBIOME PROTOCOL REGIME

In order to maximize the effectiveness of the Microbiome Protocol, the subject should consume a pristine quality of highly bio-available proteins, consume foods rich in anti-inflammatory properties, and consume healthy fats, a regimen with significant reduction in the consumption of refined carbohydrates derived from simple sugars with a low glycemic index is also recommended. It is, however, important to state, in our carb-fearing society, that not all carbs are created equally. The body does require carbohydrates for energy, and a full meal should contain an adequate quantity of them. Suggestions for a healthy, balanced diet will be discussed further in-depth later in the book. For the purpose of this protocol, we recommend a diet consisting of approximately 20% carbohydrates ideal to maximize the wellness potential— especially if the consumer has health challenges. A healthy individual should stick in that range to contribute to the efficacy of the protocol. We call this the Microbiome Protocol Regimen.

The goal of this regimen is not weight loss, and it is important that these changes in diet should be done gradually. Our protein and meal recommendations are geared toward maximizing protein and nutrient absorption rather than deprivation. It is critical that this change in dietary regimen is achieved in a progressive way without withdrawing carbohydrates too abruptly, in order to avoid weight loss and be supportive of lean muscle mass.

By creating this dietary change and feeding the supportive systems of all three brains, the Microbiome Protocol Regimen enhances the effectiveness of the Microbiome Protocol. This nutritional plan is based on increasing data that demonstrate the utility of high-quality-protein, low-carbohydrate regimes that avoid simple sugars and have low glycemic indexes.

THE MICROBIOME PROTOCOL REGIMEN 20/60/20

The basis of a 20/60/20 regimen is based on the needs of the general population. Please consult with your healthcare professional to customize a program specific to your health and nutritional requirements. Please note that if your health care professional has recommended a ketogenic diet, the 20/60/20 regime would not apply. In this case, please refer to the Ketogenic Diet, which you can find at www.ketogenicdiet.org.

The Microbiome Protocol Regimen is based ideally on a daily caloric consumption of the following proportions:

1. 20% of calories should come from complex carbohydrates with a low glycemic index

2. 60% of calories should come from high-quality protein sources

3. 20% of calories should come from healthy fats

Keep in mind that carbohydrates contain four calories per gram and proteins contain four calories per gram; however, fat contains nine calories per gram. For example, if a person is consuming a 2,000-calorie-per-day diet, 400 calories from carbohydrates (this equals 100 grams of carbohydrates), 400 calories from fat (this equals 44.44 grams of fat), and 60% of the total daily consumption of calories from a good protein source (this equals 1,200 calories from high-quality protein, or 300 grams of protein). Consult with your nutritionist or healthcare professional to determine the total daily caloric intake that is right for you.

BE A FORENSIC LABEL READER

Don't just look at the carbohydrate content, especially when certain products contain artificial sweeteners. When choosing carbohydrates, it's important to choose ones that are low glycemic. As previously stated, carbohydrates give us energy. The wrong type of carbohydrates can, however, lead us down the wrong health path. Educate yourself. Find the optimal types of carbohydrates to maximize the protocol.

GLYCEMIC INDEX AND GLYCEMIC LOAD

Every food has a glycemic index and a glycemic load. The glycemic index is tested using a selection of individuals consuming the particular food containing the carbohydrates. Once the food is consumed by the individual, insulin response is tested and recorded, giving a Glycemic Index of 0-100. Foods that receive scores under 55 are considered low glycemic. Also note that just because a food tests low glycemic, this does not always mean that it is truly healthy. Many low-glycemic foods contain artificial sweeteners such as aspartame, sucralose, and saccharin, which should be avoided at all cost. These artificial sweeteners have been studied and have been proven to negatively impact gut flora.

It is important to state that for best adherence of The Microbiome Protocol and Regimen, sticking to consuming low-glycemic foods is best. Having a low-glycemic load is important as well, as not all foods have been assessed by a third-party testing facility. According to the resource below, it is important to consider the amount of carbohydrates, protein and dietary fiber that are contained in the food to obtain the glycemic load. The glycemic load accounts for the portion and fiber content—whereas the glycemic index does not. You can check out some very informative websites that can calculate the approximate glycemic load for a food. Here is one we have used to plug in a variety of different foods: http://nutritiondata.self.com/topics/glycemic-index

They recommend the following equation:

Glycemic Load is calculated this way:

GL = GI/100 x Net Carbs

(Net Carbs are equal to the Total Carbohydrates minus Dietary Fiber). Therefore, you can control your glycemic response by consuming low-GI foods and/or by restricting your intake of carbohydrates." You can also manipulate load by eating foods rich in fiber. Prebiotic fiber is more critical, as the fibers contained slow the release of glucose in the food.[39]

PROTEINS: 60% of our daily intake should be coming from clean protein. What does that look like for meals?

---

39. http://nutritiondata.self.com/topics/glycemic-index#ixzz3Xorkqj7S

Dr. Ruggiero and his team recommend spreading protein consumption throughout the day in five small meals. Each meal should contain a generous source of protein and vegetables. Protein sources are listed below. Supplemental healthy starches may be included at minimal levels. Refined carbohydrates should be avoided.

LEAN ANIMAL PROTEIN SOURCES:

- Chicken
- Turkey
- Seafood
- Eggs
- Pork
- Undenatured New Zealand whey protein

VEGAN SOURCES:

- Peas
- Chickpea
- Fermented Non-GMO Soy
- Non-GMO Tofu
- Raw Nuts (almonds, cashews)/also a healthy fat
- Hemp seeds
- Beans
- Quinoa
- Plant-based protein shakes (multi-plant sources, non-soy, low glycemic, prebiotic fiber)

HEALTHY FATS

Among the fats choose those with the highest anti-inflammatory properties, such as coconut oil, hemp oil, flaxseed oil, and extra-virgin oil, and use them liberally. Oils containing medium-chain triglycerides are always preferred.

Low-carb, high-protein nutrition is essential to achieve the best responses from the neuro-protective, immunotherapeutic approach described below—in other words, to achieve daily optimal health.

Before we present a suggested daily menu, we wanted to clarify the types of supplemental protein that we recommend. As stated in earlier chapters of this book, we have an epic problem with lack of nutrients and trace minerals in our food supply. With this knowledge, we want to be extremely specific when it comes to any supplements. In each of the lean animal protein and vegan protein sources, we listed a protein shake or powder to incorporate into one's daily plan. It is critical that you incorporate a protein that contains trace minerals and nutrients into your diet that will feed your macrophages (the soldiers of your immune system) and ultimately feed your 2nd and 3rd brains.

Dr. Ruggiero recommends using a shake that contains 24-36 grams of undenatured New Zealand whey protein. For best absorption, it is recommended that this protein not contain calcium *caseinate* or lactose as it is essentially a raw protein that ensures that your digestive enzymes are intact.

2014 DR. RUGGIERO MAKES A HUGE DISCOVERY

For years Dr. Ruggiero has been using a particular undenatured New Zealand whey protein in his clinics across Europe. However, while speaking at Autism One in May, 2014, Dr. Ruggiero discovered a different, greatly-enhanced version of an undenatured New Zealand whey protein that was in his words a "Game Changer." Dr. Ruggiero immediately began extensive research on this newly discovered whey protein.

It is well established that high-protein/low-carbohydrate nutritional plans are very effective in health management as well as in the nutritional approach to a number of diseases ranging from cancer to autism.[40] These nutritional plans have been designated with different names, such as ketogenic, paleo or caveman diets. They have in common the need to increase the consumption of proteins while decreasing or even abolishing the consumption of carbohydrates.

40. Redox Biology 2 (2014) 963–970. Bozzetti F, Zupec-Kania B, Toward a cancer-specific diet, Clinical Nutrition (2015), http://dx.doi.org/10.1016/j.clnu.2015.01.013. Also see the potential therapeutic use of the ketogenic diet in autism spectrum disorders. Napoli E, Dueñas N, Giulivi C. Front Pediatr. 2014 Jun 30; 2:69. Doi: 10.3389/fped.2014.00069. ECollection 2014.

WHY IS PROTEIN SO CRITICAL TO MAXIMIZING OUR QUALITY-OF-LIFE?

Proteins may be the single most important molecules that a human being needs.

Did you know that our body contains approximately 15,000 different proteins?

If you were to drain all of the fluid out of the human body, you would find that approximately 50% of the dry weight of our bodies is made up of proteins. Proteins perform many critical functions in our bodies.

These includes the following:

NUTRIENT DELIVERY: First and foremost proteins are responsible for the delivery of nutrients to our cells. This is critically important for the efficient delivery of the nutritional foundations of life.

OXYGEN TRANSPORT: The delivery of oxygen in our blood-supply is vital for living.

HORMONES: Proteins enable us to move as human beings.

THE REPAIR AND REBUILDING OF OUR CELLS: Proteins are responsible for the genetic codes in our DNA. Later, we will talk about how the job of the food we eat is to communicate genetic information to our genes. Without protein this genetic information cannot be transferred.

ENZYMES: Enzymes are made from proteins and proteins are the key building blocks of muscles and bones.

WHAT HAPPENS WHEN WE INGEST PROTEIN

As we eat protein our bodies then have to break it down into individual amino acids in a process called *protein digestion*.

In laymen's terms, this process involves your body pulling the protein you consume (note: visualize multiple strands of pearls) apart into individual amino acids. Then the body has to put it all back together like reconstruction in a sense. This process of reconstruction of our body is called *body protein synthesis*. It is the reconstruction process of the amino acids rebuilding us from muscles, to bones, to our brains and all of the rest of us. This reconstruction process is going on continuously.

THE PROBLEM WITH LOW-PROTEIN DIETS

Low-protein diets that might focus on eating mainly fruits and vegetables are lacking in amino acids and therefore inhibit your maximum potential for building the best and healthiest body possible. This is why our colleagues place such high premiums on the best proteins for our patients.

Because plant-based diets often contain more sugars and carbohydrates, when consuming a vegan shake, for example, make sure it contains more than one source of vegetable protein in order to get close to the full complement of 20 amino acids the body requires.

Dr. Ruggiero explains, below, the other important roles that proteins play in our diets:

Remember, a protein is composed of approximately 300 amino acids like a string of pearls. However, when you eat a protein, first it is digested, that is where each amino acid is separated from the others and each is absorbed individually.

Then, the body uses the amino acids that have been absorbed to do three things:

1. Build body proteins, which is called Net Protein Utilization (NPU). This is the amount of amino acids that are actually absorbed by our cells and the amount that is not utilized are actually toxins to the body.

    It is critically important to understand that there is a very wide variance of "Net Protein Utilization" from different sources of Protein, be they animal or vegetable protein sources. We will cover NPU in much greater detail a little later in this chapter.

2. Convert the amino acids into glucose to provide energy.

3. Convert them into catabolites, i.e. waste products like creatinine or urea (toxins) that have to be eliminated through the kidneys and liver.

If you eat 100 grams of meat, assuming that it is all protein, the amino acids contained in those 100 grams of meat proteins will be utilized to build 30 grams of body proteins and 70 grams will be partially converted into glucose and partially into catabolites (toxins).

Clearly, amino acids are the building blocks of life that make everything in our bodies work.

HOW AMINO ACIDS WORK

Amino acids are like the letters of the alphabet. There are 20 amino acids that exist. There are two categories of amino acids. One is made up of 9 essential amino acids and the other of approximately 11 other amino acids. Some of these are made in our bodies, but the majority must be obtained from our diet.

Consider each amino acid as a letter. If you put them next to each other you form words. These words, made by letters, are the proteins. Each protein is made (on average) of 300 letters (that is by 300 amino acids). The sequence of the letters (amino acids) is different in different words. In the realm of proteins, the sequence of amino acids is responsible for the function and identity of the protein. The instructions to assemble the amino acids into proteins are contained in the genes. The human DNA contains 22,000 genes and some of them do not specify proteins. This means that one's human proteins are around 15,000. It is as if in your vocabulary you have no more than 15,000 words, each word composed of 300 letters arranged in different sequences. Each one of these words means something different: that is to say that each protein performs a different function.

For example, you eat a hamburger. It is made of cow meat. Further, the meat is made of bovine proteins that are different from human proteins, just as words in English are different from words in Italian. They have the same meaning, but the *sequence* of the letters is different. For example, the word "book" in Italian is "libro." In both languages the letters of the alphabet are the same 20 (a b c d …), but they are arranged in different sequences (book vs libro). The amino acids of a cow are the same amino acids of a man (leucine, glycine, alanine …), but they are arranged in different sequences. In your stomach and in your gut you digest the cow proteins. In other words you separate each amino acid from the other. In essence you are separating each letter. You also absorb each amino acid separately.

Next, your body uses those amino acids to build human proteins that are made by the same 20 amino acids that the cow has, but in a different sequence. It's as if you take words written in Italian, separate the letters, and then use those letters to *translate the words* into English. You will not use them all and you will be left with some letters that you cannot incorporate into English words. These are the amino acids that are not used for body protein synthesis.

This complex scientific analysis of the amount of amino acids absorbed and thus leaving the balance as waste (toxins) is called Net Protein Utilization (NPU). What will you do with those letters that you do not use to build English words? Part of them you burn to produce energy, part are discarded. Amino acids that come from that hamburger and are not used to build human proteins are partially used to provide energy (calories, mainly through their conversion into glucose through the process of gluconeogenesis), and partially are waste products (toxins).

Let's assume that you know exactly which word in English you want to write (for example, book). You take only those four letters and your letter (nitrogen) utilization will be 100%. Now, you have to take the letters that you have introduced under the form of Italian words (due Kg di buon cibo). You can use only 4 of those letters to form the English word "book". The other 9 letters are not used. Your letter (nitrogen) utilization is less than 30%. If you introduce the Master Amino Acid Pattern that is made exactly to match the human protein, it is as if you took exactly the letters that you needed to form your English words (your human proteins).

In the simplest of terms, the higher the NPU of any protein you are consuming will enhance what amino acids can do for you body.

This is because the more amino acids you have available to your genes and cells the more efficiently those amino acids can carry out all of their functions. My goal has always been to find proteins with the highest possible NPU. My scientific calculations made it clear to me that these enhanced shakes had approximately 91% of the amino acids that you need to build human proteins and only 9% waste. This was an astounding result.

This for me was truly another "Eureka Moment." We now had rock-solid scientific proof. As a result of my exhaustive analysis of these enhanced undenatured New Zealand whey protein shakes, I discovered they yielded the highest Net Protein Utilization of any protein source I had ever tested. These included animal, vegetable and the shakes I had used for years from New Zealand.

None of these protein sources were anywhere close to the NPU of these newly discovered enhanced *super shakes*. The discovery of these enhanced *super shakes* as we call now, in my opinion, will have untold positive results for all of us. These *super shakes* are a must for those who are healthy and especially for those facing medical challenges.

THE SECRET TO THIS HIGH
NET-PROTEIN UTILIZATION

It was also now clear to me why these New Zealand enhanced shakes were so extraordinarily high in this critical measurement of Net Protein Utilization.

In my analysis of these super shakes I realized that they had been enhanced by the addition of proteases (enzymes that break the proteins apart and maximize the utilization of the amino acids with little waste). I further realized that the proteins from New Zealand we had been using and tested did not contain proteases.

This had to be the reason that they had such a low Net Protein Utilization of approximately 15% with 85% waste. It was now clear that there was only one decision for me to make. That decision was to immediately begin to share these newly discovered enhanced shakes with everyone. This would include first and foremost my patients, family, friends and colleagues.

What else did my analysis reveal? As I said for years we had been using an undenatured whey protein from New Zealand (not the enhanced version I discovered in 2014). There are many reasons why we had used this undenatured New Zealand whey protein. Why is New Zealand whey protein is considered the best protein source in the world? In New Zealand, they use a low-temperature, high-filtration system. Most processing in North America use high-heat pasteurization, and thus the whey proteins are called denatured. The problem with denaturing is that the process breaks apart the protein folds that contain the branch chain amino acids. The denaturing acts like scissors to cut these critical links of the protein-to-protein called branched-chain amino acids that are like the links of a chain. This denaturing makes them much less bio available for our bodies to use. This greatly reduces their Net Protein Utilization as well.

I discovered that these enhanced un-denatured New Zealand super shakes contained proteases as well as the following additional enhancements:

PROTEASES

The proteases that must be added to the super shakes are:

- Proteases (from Aspergillus oryzae)
- Bromelain (from Ananas comosus)
- Papain (from Carica papaya)
- Acid stable protease (from Aspergillus Niger)

THE ENZYME LACTASE

The super shake should also contain the enzyme Lactase. Although these New Zealand Shakes contain almost zero lactose, the addition of the lactase will further reduce any of the remaining lactose. Thus, many people who are lactose intolerant are able to easily digest these shakes with this added enzyme.

PRE-BIOTIC FIBER PLAYS A CRITICAL ROLE

Super shakes should also contain pre-biotic fiber. I have mentioned the use of pre-biotic fiber for several reasons. First, and most importantly, it allows the body to make massive amounts of good gut bacteria that are essential to support immune health.

Secondly, the pre-biotic fiber also increases the absorption of nutrients and reduces post-prandial insulin spikes. In fact, pre-biotic fiber naturally regulates the release of glucose. This allows the use of sugar and carbohydrates to not cause insulin spikes. This is very important to producing longer-lasting energy.

Third, the super shakes contain up to 70 major minerals, minor minerals (called trace minerals) and ultratrace elements. These minerals have been called the spark plugs of life. These minerals are the co-factors for enzyme reactions, which play a crucial role in the most efficient functioning of our enzymes.

Finally, the super shake must also include vitamin D-3 and oleic acid (from olive oil). You will learn about their critical importance in magnifying the impact of The Microbiome Protocol, the food for Your Third Brain later in this book. All of these co-factors including the proteases, minerals, lactose, pre-biotic fiber, and vitamin D-3 and oleic acid, are included in this new Super Shake and should most certainly be in any shake you purchase or try to formulate yourself.

Thus these co-factors significantly enhance and improve the Super Shake we now use with all of our family, patients, friends and colleagues. For example, meat proteins are utilized for about 30%, and 70% is eliminated in the form of nitrogen catabolites that may overload the kidneys and liver. Poor-quality protein supplements are utilized only for about 20%, with 80% nitrogen catabolite toxins. In addition, poor-quality whey protein shakes, given the very low percentage of utilization for body protein synthesis, are used by the body for glyconeogenesis, a mechanism that leads to the production of glucose from proteins.

Therefore, poor-quality whey protein shakes may be harmful not only because they yield a great quantity of nitrogen catabolites that overload the kidneys and liver, but also because they nullify the very scope of ketogenic diets.

The attached chart will show you the Net Protein Utilization of other protein sources including the New Zealand undenatured whey protein shakes we had used for years until we discovered how to make this super shake we now use exclusively.

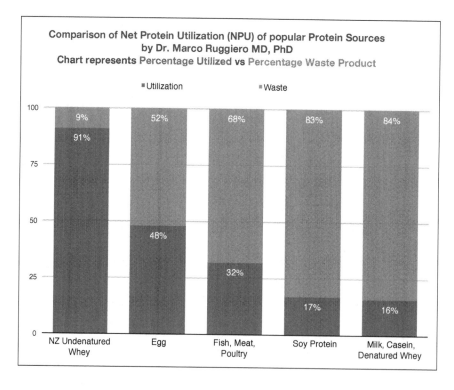

Therefore after my extensive analysis of Net Protein Utilization and the added above co-factors I came to only one conclusion and it is based totally on science. That conclusion is that every day of our lives, at least one of our meals should come from these enhanced undenatured New Zealand super shakes period.

From a scientific point of view there is no argument and only one conclusion that a researcher like myself given the evidence can come to. The conclusion is that everybody should be consuming at least one of these enhanced super shakes every day of our lives if you want to maximize your quality of life potential.

> **NOTE:** If you are sourcing or formulating your own whey protein shake, it is critical that you have a 91% Net Protein Utilization to make sure the ingestion of high protein amounts is not stressing the kidneys. We provided you with the enhanced components to create your own super shake if you have the time, expertise and patience to formulate it. That is why we have very carefully chosen these whey protein super shakes that we have discovered and utilize with our patients. The New Zealand enhanced undenatured whey protein shakes have the advantage of providing an excellent source of amino acids for body protein synthesis with no overload of kidney or liver function.

NET PROTEIN UTILIZATION ANALYSIS OF THE NUMBERS

Following is a summary by Doctor Ruggerio of one of the most significant discoveries regarding what is termed *the protein utilization* from the food we eat daily and the important differences between *protein absorption* versus *protein utilization*.

There is a lot of confusion as it relates to the meaning of Net Protein Utilization. Specifically, when analyzing this there are two very important critical differences in interpreting the analytical figures that you need to be aware of.

One analysis tells us the percentage of protein that is being absorbed into the body. At first, this information seems very important and useful. The truth, however, is that the amount of protein that is absorbed by our bodies pales in comparison to the second, and much more important analysis drawn from what is called the Net Protein Utilization. This more scientifically significant measurement references the amount of amino acids utilized from any protein source by the body.

By measuring the amino acids actually utilized by the body, the results tell scientists how much of the absorbed protein actually becomes toxic waste. These toxic waste products of absorbed protein are called nitrogen catabolites. They include toxic wastes, urea and creatine. In other words, the absorbed protein that is not utilized as amino acids, becomes toxic waste that must be eliminated through the kidneys and liver.

Net Protein Utilization Analysis of the Absorption of Protein

There are many websites that correctly state, for example, that the Net Protein Utilization measurement of absorption for eggs is 94%. In other examples they refer to the absorption of whey protein at about 92% and meat at 73%.

However their analysis of Net Protein Utilization from the percentage of the absorption of protein does not reveal the percentage of amino acids that are being utilized by the body. It's very important to know what percentage of Amino acids are converted for utilization by the body's genes and cells. Again there is a need to address the amount of toxic waste that is being produced as a result of the non-utilization of amino acids.

You can have Net Protein Utilization absorption as high as 95%. That percentage for those not trained in molecular biology seems like a very good percentage. However, the problem still exists that the amount of amino acids utilized from the protein sources tells a completely different story. The measurement of the absorption of protein does not indicate how much of that protein is converted into amino acids and how much is left as waste products or toxins (urea and creatine) that may overload the kidneys and liver.

In our analysis of the undenatured whey protein that we have used for some time (prior to our discovery of this super protein in 2014) the Net Protein Utilization of this whey protein absorption is 95% that also includes the Nitrogen Catabolites (toxins).

However when the Net Protein Utilization is scientifically measured and analyzed as the amount of the amino acids that are utilized by the body, it turns out that only 15% of the aminos can be used by the genes and cells. This means that 85% of the absorbed protein is transformed into sugars and waste that has to be eliminated by the kidneys and the liver.

The interpretation of Net Protein Utilization when looked at as 95% absorption seems great, but this percentage fails to tell the real story. A most revealing example is found in the percentage of utilization in the whey protein Dr. Ruggiero had been using. Recently he performed an analysis of it that revealed shocking results. He discovered that the Amino Acids that the body needs for so many of its key functions weighed in at only 15% utilization.

We have said in our previous books that it's not what you eat or drink. Rather it's the nutrients that your body is able to utilize that matters. The Net Protein Utilization analysis of various protein sources Dr. Ruggiero revealed represents rather than the absorption percentages the more important percentage of amino acids the body retains once the protein is absorbed and broken down through the utilization of the protein.

In conclusion, the most efficient use of protein is what is converted into the highest possible utilization of amino acids with minimal nitrogen catabolites (as I stated before, toxins that the kidneys have to deal with).

Further Findings

Another result of Dr. Ruggiero's research focused on an alternative to the shakes he had been using once he discovered his shakes had low amino acid utilization. To this end, I suggested he analyze the super shakes I have used for years. This time Dr. Ruggiero was excitedly astounded. These shakes turned to have a 91% amino acid utilization! After further analysis of other protein sources, the super shakes had no comparison of utilization close to them. Earlier we explained the critically important addition role of the proteases in these super shakes as the primary reason why the Net Protein Utilization is at 91% with only 9% as waste.

Dr. Ruggiero also took into account the other additional enhancements or co-factors added to these super shakes that included 70-plus minerals, and pre-biotic fiber. In addition, the super shakes were enhanced with vitamin D-3 and oleic acid that work synergistically to enhance the impact of the super food we have formulated for Your Third Brain.

This is why we have now switched all of our patients, friends and colleagues to these super shakes at least once a day.* I am not suggesting you not eat meat, fish or other sources of protein on a daily basis. There is no question that the consumption of one or more of these shakes per day can greatly contribute to your quality of life.

> **NOTE:** These super shakes are not currently available in Europe.

A DETOXIFICATION PROTOCOL IS ALSO OF GREAT IMPORTANCE

Based on this Net Protein Utilization information, it is apparent that our bodies are creating a great deal of waste products, even more so if we are not eating a clean and absorbable diet. This is why we highly recommend a detoxification program to assist the body in naturally removing the catabolites and other waste (toxins) that are produced through the natural process of digestion and utilization.

The enhanced super shakes discovered and analyzed by Dr. Ruggiero with The Net Protein Utilization method are the same shakes described in our other two books, *Why Diets are Failing Us* and *TDOS Syndrome and Solutions*, in the New Health Conversation Series.

ADDITIONAL CO-FACTORS MUST BE INCLUDED FOR OPTIMUM IMMUNE SYSTEM SUPPORT

An ideal formulation should also contain co-factors that synergize with known stimulators of the immune system function as well as with natural neuro-protective molecules and with natural molecules endowed with anti-cancer and anti-ageing properties. For example, oleic acid and vitamin D3, when associated in an absorbable formulation in a whey protein shake, would interact with the known vitamin D/oleic acid binding protein, conferring to this protein the above-mentioned healthy properties and establishing a powerful synergic effect.

Therefore, the New Zealand whey protein super shakes are very low in carbohydrates, containing specifically designated proteases that yield the appropriate amino acid ratios and contain co-factors such as oleic acid and vitamin D3, and may represent the ideal nutritional support in a number of health conditions.

When looking at whey protein shakes, it is valuable to be educated. As you can see, all whey protein shakes are not created equally. Many packaged products are processed in a way that much of the protein available to the body has been greatly reduced based on the Net Protein Utilization, and are not true meal replacements.

A true meal replacement is one that contains a high-quality protein, healthy carbohydrates and healthy fats. Meal replacements should range from 220-280 calories to qualify as more than a snack.

The key is to supply the body with approximately 60% of daily caloric consumption from protein, while at the same time minimizing maximizing The Net Protein Utilization factor. This way you create the least amount of Catabolites (toxins that the kidneys have to help to get rid of) which is why the super shakes play a key role in supplying a significant part of the daily needs of protein. Also, the high amount of proteases in the formulation of a super shake and the mineral detoxification mineral drink Dr. Ruggiero recommends will assist the body in getting rid of the waste created by daily ingestion of other forms of proteins that are needed to make up the total daily consumption of 60% proteins in your diet.

These other proteins have much lower Net Protein Utilization, but the waste created can be consumed because of the super shakes multiple proteases and by also utilizing the detoxification aloe vera-based mineral drink.

If you are unable to find or formulate on your own the super shake and aloe vera-based mineral drink Dr. Ruggiero utilizes with his patients and friends, you can contact us at www.yourthirdbrain.com.

BACK TO LABEL READING

Low-carb shakes can be very misleading. Many shakes tout a lowcarb solution meal replacement. It is critical to look at serving size and overall composition of the product. What seems to be low-carb may, in fact, be half of what another shake provides nutritionally in nutrients and in volume?

In essence you may need 2 ½ shakes to equal one of the shakes that we have researched and recommended.

VEGAN SHAKES WE RECOMMEND

Please note, if you will be using a vegan shake, that it is the glycemic index that matters and the ratio of carbohydrates to the amount of protein and prebiotic-fiber that matters most in this analysis. It is also critical, in our view, that the vegan shakes contain multiple sources of vegan proteins.

A vegan shake that uses pea protein as its main source of protein will be woefully short in the amino acids the body requires.

That is why vegan shakes need to have multiple sources of vegetable proteins in the end to supply the body with all the amino acids it needs to reconstruct itself.

And the vegan shakes should also contain large quantities of minerals, and trace minerals.

Use an aloe vera-based mineral drink for detoxification support as well as second-brain immune system support.

ALOE VERA-BASED MINERAL DRINK—HEALING ON MANY LEVELS

Use of an aloe vera based mineral drink is recommended for second-brain immune system support and natural detoxification. This aloe vera drink can be utilized for various beneficial purposes. Use of an aloe vera mineral drink has proven beneficial for an intermittent fasting protocol and for daily consumption.

For the confident kitchen chemists who would like to try to formulate this at home, it is important to only use the inner heart filet of the aloe plant. The gel contained in the inner heart contains very powerful polysaccharides. Polysaccharides found in the aloe gel are commonly noted for detoxification, immune support, and digestive health. Once the appropriate amount of gel is extracted from the plant, it should be carefully processed at low temperature and then spray dried to preserve the enzymes and nutrients. Be wary of any aloe vera mineral drink that touts "full-leaf" as the inclusion of the full leaf can destroy the healing properties of the polysaccharides, minerals and nutrients.

This mineral drink should also contain bilberries, blueberries and raspberries; all of which serve as great sources of antioxidants and are designed to work with all other nutrients to advance the nutritional fasting and detoxification processes.

The Microbiome Protocol Regimen, as we stated, is based on 20% carbohydrates, but this should be in conjunction with 60% of the daily caloric consumption of high-quality protein sources and 20% good fats. Note that your individual meals may not be exactly in the 20/60/20 ratio. It is your overall daily consumption totals that matter most at the end of the day.

These super shakes constitute some of the best meal replacements and are formulated to be low glycemic in nature. They are nutritionally dense, and rich in vitamins, minerals, and other beneficial phytochemicals. They also contain the beneficial eight grams of prebiotic fiber, which is critical in regulating the release of sugar while avoiding dangerous insulin spikes.

THE MICROBIOME PROTOCOL CO-COFACTORS

In addition, as we will explain in the following section, one of the most important compounds of the Microbiome Protocol is the Bravo probiotic from Bravo USA, a unique lactic ferment that contains beneficial bacteria and a wide array of live microbes and probiotics that reconstitutes the healthy core human microbiome. Mixing the Bravo with the super shakes provides a significant advantage. The super shakes work synergistically with Bravo.

Furthermore, the undenatured proteins and the protease (enzymes that break proteins down into highly absorbable peptides) in these super shakes work in synergy with the peptides and proteins deriving from the proprietary fermentation process of Bravo, and the end result is an excellent meal replacement that fits the scope of this protocol.

Divide your daily caloric intake into five mini meals with the goal of avoiding long periods of fasting. This will help you avoid insulin peaks, which weaken the immune system.

It can also be advisable to use apple cider vinegar (Braggs is an option) as a dressing in order to break biofilms.

ADDITIONAL RECOMMENDATIONS

It is also highly recommended that you add a natural destress routine such as yoga, meditation, etc. to your Microbiome Regimen. Another great addition to your regimen is a graceful aging product.

For more information on the Super Shakes, anti-stress or graceful aging technologies used by Dr. Ruggiero, please contact us at www.yourthirdbrain.com.

FOOD FOR THE THIRD BRAIN

Bravo probiotic (BP) is a proprietary array of live microbes that, during the fermentation of mammal milk and colostrum, naturally produce a number of protein peptides which support the immune system, graceful aging, and cardiac recovery. More importantly, the live microbes contained in BP reconstitute the human healthy core microbiome, which is the ultimate goal of this protocol.

The Standard American Diet consists of high-sugar, simple-carb, high-fat regimens, which are horrible for gut microbes. A regimen high in fat, sugar, and simple carbs is bad for the "healthy" gut microbes that keep us thin, and it encourages the growth of "unhealthy" microbes that make us obese.

For example, bacteria transplanted from overweight mice to thin mice make the thin mice gain weight. The relationship among genetics, the environment, and the microbiome as it relates to obesity is certainly complex. But while the genome is fixed and habits are hard to change, the microbiome is changeable. In the reverse of the mouse study described above, could microbes from thin people help obese people become healthier? Or could a nutritional supplement help healthy microbes grow?

In addition to supplying the genetic information that reconstitutes the human microbiome, most of the microbial strains contained in Bravo show per se beneficial effects of supporting a healthy immune system, and have been published in peer-reviewed studies in major medical publications. This has been shown to be an effective approach to supporting our immune system, heart health, graceful aging, and neurons.

For example, during the proprietary fermentation, the vitamin D binding protein (VDBP) that is abundant in mammal milk and colostrum is converted into the active VDBP-derived macrophage activating factor.[41]

This protocol was developed to maximize the health-promoting effects of Bravo by combining nutritional and natural approaches.

To find a Bravo health professional near you and to receive more information visit www.bravousa.com.

THE RECIPE FOR THE SUPER SHAKE

BRAVO SUPER SHAKE: THE HIGHEST QUALITY UNDENATURED PROTEINS

To prepare the "Super Shake" for an adult weighing 165 pounds, take four ounces of the BP after it has been produced and is ready to drink, and put it in a 500 ml jar.

Then, add one or two tablespoons of the BP to the super shake Dr. Ruggiero recommends.

The reason he recommends these super shake formulations is because they are poor in carbs and rich in minerals, vitamins, and prebiotic fiber that synergizes with Bravo.

This is what he is recommending and using with all of his patients in North America.

---

41. (*Nutrients.* 2013 Jul 8; 5(7):2577-89. J Neuroinflammation. 2014 Apr 17; 11:78. Anticancer Res. 2014 Jul; 34(7):3569-78. *Anticancer Drugs.* 2015 Feb; 26(2):197-209). Interestingly, one of the strains in BP, *Lactobacillus Rhamnosus* also activates macrophages (*Microbiol Immunol.* 2012 Nov; 56(11):771-81)

Then, add half a teaspoon of hemp oil and half a teaspoon of coconut oil to the super shake. Extra-virgin olive oil can also be used. A mixture of coconut and hemp oil would be ideal.

Add one teaspoon of good-quality lecithin that helps in the natural formation of liposomes.

Bring to volume (*i.e.* to 500 ml) of water.

NOTE: Grind/blend/shake very well with a blender for a few minutes until a very homogeneous smooth emulsion is produced: a liposome/ micronized emulsion is now in the jar, the contact surface of all the peptides and proteins derived from the fermentation of BP, including GcMAF, is enormously increased, and all the beneficial principles are now readily absorbable.

It is best to drink your shake slowly in order to enjoy the texture and the taste. These shakes taste really great.

This shake is one of the five meals that should be eaten. Always shake it very well before drinking; the micronized emulsion lasts only a few minutes after the shaking process has taken place as the cold water stimulates the enzyme reactions.

BRAVO AS A FOOD

If the "Super Shake" option is not feasible, prepare and drink Bravo according to the manufacturer's instructions. Take 10-120 ml (the dose depends on the body weight. 120 ml is the dose for a 75 Kg adult) per day, every day. If a person is not accustomed to dairy products, begin with a small amount (half a teaspoon) and gradually increase detoxification. Also, it is the inner filet that contains special polysaccharides, which have been studied for their ability to balance the immune system and their actions as natural detoxifiers, helping to move along biochemical processes in the liver to neutralize toxins. Many other aloe vera supplements use high heat that actually destroys the polysaccharides and other nutrients. So, where you get your aloe vera from really does matter.

In addition to the beneficial effects of utilizing only the inner heart filet of aloe vera (if you choose to formulate this on your own) and the "Mineral Suites" (that should include major minerals, micro-minerals and ultratrace elements) as a drink, it should also include bilberries, blueberries and raspberries, all of which serve as great sources of antioxidants and are designed to work with all other nutrients to advance the nutritional fasting processes.

These nutritionally dense ingredients treat the body as a whole, supplying it with massive amounts of nutrients, vitamins and the ever-so-critical "Mineral Suites."

NOW ON TO THE SAMPLE DAILY PLAN

UPON WAKE UP

Aloe Vera Mineral Drink (2-4 oz.)

BREAKFAST (MEAL 1)

Easy On-the-Go Super Shake – for sustained focus and energy

6-9 oz. purified water (preferred high pH)

> 3-4 cubes of ice
> 60-70 g New Zealand whey meal replacement powder 4 oz.
> Bravo Probiotic (see preparation instructions)
> 1t sunflower lecithin
> 1T healthy oil (hemp, flax, mct, coconut) 2 Super Minerals
> 1 Lithium Orotate

Combine all ingredients and blend on high for 20-30 seconds.

Drink shake within 10 minutes, as the enzymatic activity is critical for absorption. You may swish the shake around the mouth for best results. After enjoying this breakfast treat -avoid eating or drinking for one hour. Since many toothpaste brands contain artificial sweeteners, it is crucial that you brush your teeth prior to consuming (not after)

MORNING SNACK (MEAL 2)

2 Hard boiled eggs with cucumber slices

LUNCH (MEAL 3)

Grilled Vegetable Salad with Roasted Salmon

(4-6 oz.) protein and ½ -1 cup grilled vegetables (prepared with coconut, avocado, grapeseed oil, extra virgin olive oil)

AFTERNOON SNACK (MEAL 4)

Organic Celery with 2T raw almond butter

DINNER (MEAL 5)

Asher's Easy Stir-fry

> 2 T coconut aminos 1T gluten free tamari
>
> 1T grapeseed oil (+1 for later) 2T chili-flakes
>
> 1 lb. organic chicken breast - cut into 1" cubes 1 lb. shrimp-cleaned and deveined
>
> 1 egg - lightly scrambled
>
> 1 bunch of asparagus, cleaned and cut into 1" pieces 1 cup bean sprouts

Combine first four ingredients in a small bowl. Set aside.

Heat oil in pan on medium heat or flame. Add egg and scramble. When fully cooked, set egg aside.

Add ½ T oil to pan and Sautee chicken and shrimp until chicken is cooked through and shrimp is opaque. Add bean sprouts and asparagus and cook for an additional three minutes. Add egg and liquid to pan. Mix until sauce is thoroughly combined throughout.

DESSERT (MEAL 6)

Whey Protein Shake with a scoop of alkalizing superfood greens.

10

Mysteries of Wonder Molecules from Heparin to GcMAF

Even many centuries after Galileo, there is the tendency to build dogmas that, in time, become irrefutable truths, and are very often are critically accepted by other researchers. However, in many cases, the dogma that is often more palatably designated with words such as "widely accepted" or "universal consensus" fails to explain certain observations. In more than thirty years of research, I have been fascinated by a number of molecules whose properties challenged all that was known at that time. These molecules presented a wonderful opportunity to try to do what always excites scientists, that is to drive toward a paradigm shift and therefore challenge the dogma and propose a different hypothesis that can explain the observation.

If the scientist who challenges the "universal consensus" demonstrates that they are right, they will have opened an entire new field of knowledge. Otherwise, their career will be terminated. And the "universal consensus" is not an easy beast to defeat just because it is universal. Therefore, when a scientist embarks on such an adrenalinic enterprise, they know from the start that all the other researchers in the world will be ready to crucify them just because they rarely accept that the certainty of a dogma is put in discussion.

Thirty years ago, when I was a young, inexperienced researcher at the Laboratory of Molecular Biology of the University of Firenze, I met Dr. Simonetta Vannucchi, MD, a professor of general pathology at the same university. General pathology is a typical continental discipline that is not very common in Anglo-Saxon countries. It is based on the principles of the *Allgemeine Pathologie* (German for general pathology), a discipline that focuses on the common characteristics shared by different diseases. In fact, although diseases have different causes (aetiology) and different ways to progress (pathogenesis), they share core common features at the cellular and molecular levels. Simonetta, who was my senior, spent all her academic life investigating a single molecule, heparin, and, with my little help, she was able to discover the most important feature of this molecule, a feature that no one could even imagine.

THE MYSTERY MOLECULE HEPARIN

The name heparin derives from the word in Ancient Greek for liver, an organ in which it is found in abundance. Essentially, it is a sugar, or to be more precise, a highly sulfated glycosaminoglycan that is commonly used as an injectable anticoagulant. It is one of the strangest molecules of all, since it shows the highest negative charge density of any known biological molecule; this means that its surface is electrically charged with negative charges, just like the negative pole of a battery. Such a density of negative charges makes this molecule extremely hydrophilic; this means that this molecule is easily solubilized in water and, conversely, it should be impossible to solubilize in oily solutions.

In addition to these intriguing features, although we have large amounts of heparin circulating in our bloodstream and residing in our organs, its physiological role is still unknown. In fact, it is well assessed that endogenous heparin does not contribute to maintaining our blood fluid; that is, it does not exert a physiological anticoagulant effect (these effects are exerted by another glycosaminoglycan that is called heparan sulfate). To further corroborate this fact, it should be noticed that heparin is produced by a number of widely different species, including some invertebrates that do not have a similar blood coagulation system. Logically, the functions of endogenous heparin have to be others than inhibition of coagulation.

There are various hypotheses concerning the physiological role of heparin, and it has been proposed that, rather than anticoagulation, the main purpose of heparin is defense at sites of injuries against invading bacteria and other foreign materials. As we shall see later, not only may this hypothesis be fundamentally correct, but heparin could also help us in defending against cancer cells.

In the mid eighties, we were working on two fronts. On one side, we wanted to extract heparin from human plasma to study whether it was circulating as a single molecule or if it was associated with other molecules in plasma such as proteins; on the other side, we wanted to study its effects on cancer cells cultured *in vitro*, a type of experiment that curiously had not been performed before.

In order to characterize the molecular assembly of heparin in human plasma, we withdrew some blood from ourselves, separated the cells from the plasma by centrifugation, added some radioactive heparin to the plasma, and then extracted the molecules from the plasma with a method that is called "Folch extraction". By this method, oily lipids are separated from proteins and sugars that instead are recovered in the aqueous phase of the extraction. We had opted for this method because first, we wanted to get rid of the plasma lipids like cholesterol and triglycerides that would have hampered further purification of the material, and then study the molecules (that we presumed to be proteins) that bound the radioactive heparin. We had used radioactive heparin because we could have followed the radioactivity and, hence, the association between the heparin and candidate proteins.

Obviously, we expected that all radioactive heparin would be recovered in the aqueous phase, since again, heparin itself (radioactive labeling does not modify the chemical characteristics of any molecule) is highly hydrophilic.

MY ZEAL LED TO AN AMAZING DISCOVERY WITH HEPARIN

In those days, we measured radioactivity with an instrument that was called a liquid scintillator and required a laborious preparation of the samples. Since I was the youngest of the group, I had been given the lackluster task of preparing the samples for counting the radioactivity, and I had taken my assignment very seriously, so seriously that, in an excess of zeal, I decided to prepare for radioactive counting of all the samples, including the oily phases where, according to logic, no heparin should have ever been present.

And, given these premises, it is easy to understand the astonishment that caught me when, in the solitary and quite unhealthy room of the liquid scintillator, I saw that radioactive counts were read by the instrument in the oily phase. I checked several times to see whether I had misplaced the samples inside the instrument, but there had been no errors, and the amazing reality was developing in front of my eyes with the impartial mechanical "tick-tock" of the old electric machine attached to the liquid scintillator.

THE IMPOSSIBLE BECOMES POSSIBLE

This serendipitous observation was repeated many times, at a detriment to our blood pools, and every time, we were able to recover heparin from the oily phase. This meant only one thing; defying all rules of electrology, the most negatively charged molecule in the organic universe was associated with the hydrophobic lipids, just as if oil and water could uniformly and spontaneously mix. We worked at this project with renewed enthusiasm for months until we decided to submit our results and interpretations to one of the most prestigious scientific journal of those days: the *Biochemical Journal*, printed in the United Kingdom. In this paper, we described how the impossible was real and how heparin bound to phosphatidylcholine (also known as lecithin), the most abundant phospholipid in our bodies, since it constitutes that membrane of all of our cells.

This discovery of ours was a true paradigm shift and prompted us to rethink the physiological role of heparin. We, like all other researchers in the field, had thought that the role of heparin was somehow associated with maintaining the good health of the cardiovascular system, misguided in this assumption by the well-known pharmacological use of heparin. But now, we had to hypothesize other roles, and we immediately went to perform the experiments on the cancerous cells that we had in our cultures *in vitro*.

It took us six years before we could finally prove that heparin actually directly inhibited the proliferation of cancer cells *in vitro*, thus opening new perspectives for the use of heparin as an anti-cancer agent.

> **NOTE:** These experiments were done in vitro which is in a Petri dish outside the body, and in no way is to be implied that this is a cure for cancer, as it is not. It is the clinical observation of Dr. Ruggiero and his team who continue to pursue research with Heparin along with other researchers around the world as a possible tool in conjunction with proven medical treatments and protocols. The results have inspired researchers to do a great deal more research on Heparin's possible benefits as a protective molecule.

Today the role of heparin in cancer is very well recognized, even though there have been no attempts to translate these features that we had discovered decades ago into actual anticancer drugs. In a recent review published in 2015 in the Annals of Medicine, Franchini and Mannucci write "… heparins may improve overall survival of cancer patients by influencing directly the tumor biology."[42]

> **NOTE:** Again, it is important for the reader to be cautioned that the findings may improve the survival rates, but more study needs to be done on this possibility. These observations are just that and are not to be in any way misconstrued as a statement that this is a cure for cancer.

---

42. *Annals of Medicine*, 2015; Early Online: 1–6 © 2015 Informa UK, Ltd. ISSN 0785-3890 print/ISSN 1365-2060 online DOI: 10.3109/07853890.2015.1004361.

In the following years, we tried to elucidate the molecular mechanisms that are responsible for these anticancer properties of heparin and that enable heparin to perform a novel type of anticancer surveillance on our bodies. In fact, we had previously demonstrated that heparin binds to the surface of cells, possibly through association with phosphatidylcholine and, after binding, it is carried inside the cells or, as we say in scientific terms, it is "internalized."[43]

In the same years when we were performing our experiments on heparin and cancer cells *in vitro*, it was demonstrated by other researchers that heparin bound to histones (the proteins that keep the DNA in the cell nucleus properly folded).[44] This type of interaction was not surprising, since heparin has a number of negative charges on its surface, whereas histones are positive charges. The novel observation, in this case, was to have demonstrated that heparin could be carried inside the cells, a feature that was not deemed possible before we had demonstrated it.

At this point, it was easy to conclude that the binding of heparin to the DNA of cancer cells altered the expression of the genes of these cells; these are complicated words to say that most likely, heparin disturbed the functioning of the DNA of cancer cells in such a way that cancer cells were no longer able to replicate, as we had demonstrated in our paper of 1991. It is well known that cancer cells are essentially unable to repair DNA damage, and this inability is at the base of

43. *Biochem Biophys Res Commun.* 1986 Oct 15;140(1):294-301. *Internalization and metabolism of endogenous heparin by cultured endothelial cells.* Vannucchi S, Pasquali F, Chiarugi V, Ruggiero M.

44. *Biochemistry.* 1989 Apr 18;28(8):3518-25. *Heparin binds to intact mononucleosomes and induces a novel unfolded structure.* Brotherton TW, Jagannadham MV, Ginder GD.

all conventional anticancer therapies such as radiation therapy or chemotherapy.[45] Therefore, it can be hypothesized that heparin might selectively kill the cancer cells and not do harm to the normal cells, since the latter can potentially repair the damage inflicted by heparin to their histone/DNA assembly.

> **NOTE:** This is an observation and has to be analyzed with more extensive research. This is a hypothesis which demonstrates that investing more research time and money into the role of Heparin is worthwhile by researchers. Our purpose here is to make you aware of cutting edge scientific observations and investigation that may and we want to emphasize may have benefits in the future.

GCMAF ANOTHER MYSTERY MOLECULE IS DISCOVERED

Interestingly, this hypothesis, that selectivity in killing cancer cells corresponds to the absence of side effects should these concepts be translated into actual anticancer therapies, is shared by another component of our body and our diet, oleic acid, the healthy fatty acid of olive oil, whose beneficial properties have been known to mankind for thousands of years.

In fact, it appears that oleic acid, when it is physiologically associated with carrier proteins, has been observed in studies to selectively kill the cancer cells. In a recent paper describing the association between oleic acid and lactalbumin, a milk protein, the authors explicitly write: "α-Lactalbumin (α-LA) can bind oleic acid (OA)

---

45. For a recent review on this topic, please see: Trends Genet. 2014 Aug;30(8):326-39. doi: 10.1016/j.tig.2014.06.003. Epub 2014 Jul 10. *Cancer-specific defects in DNA repair pathways as targets for personalized therapeutic approaches.* Dietlein F, Thelen L, Reinhardt HC.

to form HAMLET-like complexes, which exhibited **highly selective anti-tumor activity in vitro and in vivo.**[46] It is worth noticing that these complexes between milk proteins and oleic acid are highly represented in the fermented milk product that we defined as "the third brain in a dessert cup".

NOTE: This third brain dessert cup or super food is not a cure or a treatment for any disease. This third brain dessert cup, as we call it, contains ingredients that are beneficial in supporting our immune system as well as supporting the goal of contributing to maximizing our wellness potential. These statements have not been evaluated by the FDA, and in no way is this a substitute for proper medical advice, procedures or protocols.

MYSTERY AND DISCOVERY OF GCMAF MOLECULE

Now that the mystery of heparin had been solved, we could confront another mystery molecule, the Gc protein-derived Macrophage Activating Factor or GcMAF, a molecule that has been the target of research as well as of hot arguments and criticisms for the past twenty-five years.

I had begun working on the role of macrophage activators since 1990, when I was a visiting scientist at the National Cancer Institute of the National Institutes of Health in Bethesda, MD, USA. Macrophages are cells of our immune system that work as sentinels that recognize and neutralize cells infected by viruses and bacteria, as well as cancer cells. Therefore, we want to keep these sentinels of that army that

---

46. *Biochim Biophys Acta.* 2014 Apr 4; 1841(4):535-43. doi: 10.1016/j.bbalip.2013.12.008. Epub 2013 Dec 22.
Bovine lactoferrin binds oleic acid to form an anti-tumor complex similar to HAMLET.
Fang B, Zhang M, Tian M, Jiang L, Guo HY, Ren FZ.

is our immune system in the best possible state of fitness, well fed and well equipped so that they can perform their task with maximal efficiency. In addition, it is only logical to hypothesize that if we can further empower these cells, the entire functionality of the immune system will improve and, in particular, the surveillance against cancer cells will also, the so-called anti-cancer immune surveillance.

MACROPHAGE STIMULATING FACTOR

With these goals very clear in our minds, we begun to study a particular protein called Macrophage Stimulating Factor in human leukemia cells, and the results of our studies were deemed so import-ant as to be published in one of the most, if not the most, presti-gious journals in the field of science: the *Proceedings of the National Academy of Sciences of the USA*.

Here we are providing you with the first page of our article on macrophage stimulation published in 1990 in PNAS that has been widely endorsed in the scientific community.

At about the same time, several researchers were studying another protein, somehow related, that stimulated macrophages and whose production was thought to be reduced in cancer patients as well as in patients with a variety of chronic diseases. This protein had been des-ignated with different names that reflected its multiplicity of effects. Since it was known that it binds vitamin D, some researchers had called it vitamin D binding protein-derived Macrophage Activating Factor or DBP-MAF. However, since it was also called Gc globulin, other researchers coined the lucky name GcMAF, which stands for

Gc globulin (or Gc protein)-derived Macrophage Activating Factor. This latter acronym evidently was more palatable and stuck.

This protein has been used in a variety of experimental systems and in a few clinical studies, and it showed remarkable properties that, however, were very difficult to explain. The variety of effects observed ranged from the obvious stimulation of macrophages to direct inhibition of cancer cell proliferation, inhibition of angiogenesis (the process that enables the tumor to form new blood vessels that bring oxygen and nutrients to the growing tumor), and protection againstneurotoxicity and, therefore, possible benefits in neurodegenerative and neurodevelopmental disorders.

GCMAF UNREALISTIC CLAIMS

This variety of effects, along with some unrealistic claims that this protein could have been the cure for a number of diseases, led many skeptics to conclude that it was another type of snake oil devoid of any real beneficial property. We had begun working with GcMAF in 2009, when we were studying the so-called vitamin D axis. In fact, vitamin D, a molecule that is more a hormone than a *bona fide* vitamin, exerts all its actions in our bodies thanks to the interaction with two proteins that are its intracellular receptor (the vitamin D receptor or VDR), and the vitamin D binding protein (also termed Gc protein, as I have described above).

Our first paper on the association between variations of the VDR and metastatic breast cancer was published in 1998 (*Vitamin D receptor gene polymorphism is associated with metastatic breast cancer.)*[47] And more than ten years later, we begun to wonder whether GcMAF, another component of the vitamin D axis, was also involved in human cancer. Therefore, we conducted a number of experiments that led to the publication of a significant number of peer-reviewed papers on the issue, making our research group the most proficient in this particular field of science that is often designated with the noun "immunotherapy".

IMMUNOTHERAPY

Immunotherapy, as you will learn in the next chapter, was discovered almost 130 years ago by Dr. William Caley in New York City and is now the focus of much new research. The concept is that stimulating the immune system helps to protect the body before it gets out of balance (homeostasis). Immunotherapy, 130 years later, is now being rediscovered and reintroduced in conjunction with conventional medical procedures and protocols by more and more medical researchers, health professionals and allopathic physicians.

In 2011, for the very first time, we demonstrated that GcMAF and heparin interacted in that particular phenomenon that is the cancer cell-stimulated angiogenesis (*Gc protein-derived macrophage-activating factor (GcMAF) stimulates CAMP formation in human mononuclear cells and inhibits angiogenesis in chick embryo chorionallantoic membrane assay.)*[48] To our great surprise, the two molecules that have had a prominent role in my scientific career,

47. Ruggiero M, Pacini S, Aterini S, Fallai C, Ruggiero C, Pacini P. *Oncol Res.* 1998; 10(1):43-6.

48. Pacini S, Morucci G, Punzi T, Gulisano M, Ruggiero M. Cancer Immunol Immunother. 2011 Apr; 60(4):479-85.

heparin and GcMAF, showed a molecular interaction that would have led to some interesting developments.

Soon thereafter, in 2012, we demonstrated that GcMAF inhibited the proliferation of human breast cancer cells in culture and that this effect was superimposable to that of vitamin D itself *(Effects of vitamin D-binding protein-derived macrophage-activating factor on human breast cancer cells.)*[49] A few months later, we elucidated the mechanism of action at the molecular level, and we found that the same variations (polymorphisms) of the VDR that we had observed in metastatic breast cancer were also responsible for the effects of GcMAF in human macrophages.[50]

Thus, we now had four molecules that were interacting with each other: the GcMAF protein, the VDR, the vitamin D, and our old friend, heparin. It was only one year later, in 2013, when we discovered that another molecule was also participating in this multimolecular assembly, and this molecule was nothing less than oleic acid, a molecule known to mankind for thousands of years for its beneficial effects (a novel role for a major component of the vitamin D axis): vitamin D binding protein-derived macrophage activating factor induces human breast cancer cell apoptosis through stimulation of macrophages.[51]

49. Pacini S, Punzi T, Morucci G, Gulisano M, Ruggiero M. Anticancer Res. 2012 Jan;32(1):45-52.

50. *Effect of paricalcitol and GcMAF on angiogenesis and human peripheral blood mononuclear cell proliferation and signaling.* Pacini S, Morucci G, Punzi T, Gulisano M, Ruggiero M, Amato M, Aterini S. J Nephrol. 2012 Jul-Aug; 25(4):577-81.

51. Thyer L, Ward E, Smith R, Fiore MG, Magherini S, Branca JJ, Morucci G, Gulisano M, Ruggiero M, Pacini S. Nutrients. 2013 Jul 8; 5(7):2577-89.

And, finally, between 2014 and 2015, we discovered two other important properties of these multimolecular complexes: their ability to protect human neurons and glial cells from the damage inflicted by heavy metals, and their ability to maintain a healthy circulatory system through the production of a gas called nitric oxide.

In two papers published in 2015, we demonstrated that these complexes of GcMAF, oleic acid, vitamin D, VDR and glycosamino-glycans were able to protect the human neurons and the human glial cells (which form the connective tissue in our first brain) from the damage inflicted by a heavy metal commonly used in anti-cancer chemotherapy, oxaliplatin.[52] These papers of ours open a new perspective in the integrative therapy of cancer, because they demonstrate how conventional chemotherapy can be accompanied by immunotherapy, minimizing the side effects and maximizing the therapeutic effects.

In another paper, published in 2014 in the journal *Anticancer Research,*[53] we demonstrated that these complexes stimulated the formation of a gas, nitric oxide, that is essential for the maintenance of the functionality of our cardiovascular system and also shows very promising anticancer properties.

---

52. Effects of oxaliplatin and oleic acid Gc-protein-derived macrophage-activating factor on murine and human microglia. Branca JJ, Morucci G, Malentacchi F, Gelmini S, Ruggiero M, Pacini S. J Neurosci Res. 2015 Mar 18. Doi: 10.1002/jnr.23588. Gc-protein-derived macrophage activating factor counteracts the neuronal damage induced by oxaliplatin. Morucci G, Branca JJ, Gulisano M, Ruggiero M, Paternostro F, Pacini A, Di Cesare Mannelli L, Pacini S. Anticancer Drugs. 2015 Feb; 26(2):197-209.

53. *Oleic Acid, deglycosylated vitamin D-binding protein, nitric oxide: a molecular triad made lethal to cancer.* Ruggiero M, Ward E, Smith R, Branca JJ, Noakes D, Morucci G, Taubmann M, Thyer L, Pacini S. Anticancer Res. 2014 Jul;34(7):3569-78.

NOTE: This is exciting research but keep in mind, this is in the laboratory in a Petri dish and not in-vivo (inside the body). As we have stated, more research must be done. The reader again needs to be aware that this is the scientific process of research that may prove to be useful weapon alongside established and proven medical protocols, drugs and therapies.

NOTE 2: A note of caution. More research has to be conducted. Although this research has shown promise in vitro (in a Petri dish) it in no way is a cure for any disease. This is not meant to be seen as a substitute for conventional medical treatments. The published results are promising and are worthy of more study, but more research is necessary

What is most amazing is that these multimolecular (or supramolecular) complexes endowed with such interesting biological properties are naturally present in certain types of foods, such as those that I have described when dealing with the possibility of reconstituting the healthy core human microbiome in a dessert cup. And this consideration led us to the experiments that we are performing today.

In fact, as scientists, we always have to have two perspectives in our research: the analytical and the synthetic. In other words, we have to study biological phenomena by looking simultaneously at the single tree and at the forest as a whole. If we do not adopt both approaches, we run the risk of severely misinterpreting our observation. Therefore, having observed that these multi-molecular complexes, whether recreated in a laboratory or naturally present in a fermented milk product, exerted a number of functions, now we had to establish which part of the complex exerted which function. It is worth remembering that these complexes, in particular when in their physiological matrix (that is, the food termed "microbiome in a cup"), exert a large number of effects that could be potentially exploited in future treatment approaches in conjunction with conventional medical approaches in neurology, neuro-development, anti-ageing and cardiology. Therefore, for researchers, it is of utmost importance to assess which molecule is responsible for what, so as to develop specific approaches aimed at specific wellness challenges.

To our greatest surprise and after years of experiments on the GcMAF protein, we eventually discovered that all the biological properties attributed to this multifaceted molecule were not due to the protein itself, but rather to the molecules that it carried. In other words, the GcMAF protein is simply a carrier that can be substituted for by any other molecule with the same physico-chemical characteristics. This realization came as a shock, since we had always thought that the properties of GcMAF, described by hundreds of scientists for more than twenty years, were due to the particular molecular conformation of the protein.

But it was just the careful study of such a molecular conformation that led us to conclude that in reality, GcMAF is only the carrier, like a taxi that carries surgeons to the hospital. The brand or the color of the taxi is irrelevant as long as it can carry the doctors to the place where they can perform their jobs and save lives. And if taxis are not available, any other type of transportation will achieve the same goal, and the doctors will still be able to save lives. In molecular terms, this meant that thirty years after our paradigm shift in the field of heparin, we had prompted another paradigm shift, this time in the field of immunotherapy. We had demonstrated that the taxi called GcMAF can be substituted with other vehicles, other molecules, which can perform the same task with greater efficiency.

In summary, our observational studies have demonstrated that this dessert in a cup is simply supplying the body with entirely naturally occurring molecules that are created as part of our natural immune system at birth. We have demonstrated, at the very least, that these natural molecules support our immune system, cardiovascular health, neurons and generally a better quality of life.

Just when this book was going into the press, exciting news confirming our observation was announced. Researchers at the University of Virginia School of Medicine determined that the brain is directly connected to the immune system through lymphatic vessels that had not been characterized before. These small vessels are located in the proximity of the meninges, the protective layers that envelope the brain and participate in the exchanges of molecules between the brain and the blood and lymphatic circulation. The researchers at the University of Virginia immediately recognized that such an observation has the potential to change our approach to a number of neuro-developmental and neuro-degenerative disorders ranging from autism to Alzheimer, from multiple sclerosis to amyotrophic lateral sclerosis. In fact, all these diseases are characterized by a dysfunction of the immune system inside the brain and by widespread inflammation. Therefore, this observation indicates that cells of the immune system, such as macrophages, can actually penetrate the brain, a notion that was completely ignored until now. And, these observation can also explain the excellent therapeutic effects that have been observed by treating patients with autism or neuro-degenerative diseases with the nutritional immunotherapeutic approach based on GcMAF described in the other chapters of this book. In fact, it is now possible to hypothesize that macrophages activated by

GcMAF recirculate from the blood to the brain through these newly discovered vessels and participate in the healing processes that lead to the significant improvements described by the hundreds of therapists who are using this approach. In addition, these recent observation confirm the oneness of the brain inside our head, the gut, the immune system and the microbiome (i.e. the third brain). It can now be safely assumed that these four organs, previously intended as distinct, are in actuality different anatomical part of the same organ, the third brain, that is the organ that directs the functions most important for our life.

NOTE: None of these statements have been evaluated by the Food and Drug Administration. The dessert, as we call it, in a cup is not a cure or treatment for any disease. Therefore, none of these scientific observations should in any way substituted for sound medical advice from health practitioners and/or allopathic physicians.

11

The Use of Ultrasound
for the Third Brain

This chapter shares Dr. Ruggiero's observational published studies on the use of ultrasonography with his patients. In many of his patients, it has greatly enhanced their quality of life, especially for those with significant medical challenges.

> **NOTE:** None of the statements in this chapter have been evaluated by the Food and Drug Administration. These observations and published studies are simply Dr. Ruggiero's and his colleagues' and are not cures for any disease or illness. They are in no way substitutes for conventional medical practices. It is highly recommended that you consult with your health professional or allopathic physician who are licensed and trained in the use of ultrasonography before acting on any of these observations.

DR. RUGGIERO

The Gospel of John begins with the famous verse: "In the beginning was the Word, and the Word was with God, and the Word was God". In Greek it reads:Ἐν ἀρχῇ ἦν ὁ λόγος, καὶ ὁ λόγος ἦν πρὸς τὸν θεόν, καὶ θεός ἦν ὁ λόγος.En archē ēn ho Lógos, kai ho Lógos ēn pros ton Theón, kai Theós ēn ho Lógos.

The true meaning of the Greek word "Logos" continues to be a source of vigorous debate among Bible translators, and although I studied ancient Greek for five years in college, I have no competence whatsoever to contribute to this debate. However, here I wish to concentrate on the literal meaning of the word "Logos" that, as it is always translated in English, means "word". What is a word? If we use Derrida's technique and we wish to understand the meaning of the word "word", we have to first ask ourselves what it is in terms of fundamental particles, and this is relatively easy. A word is nothing else than a sound, and a sound is the transmission of mechanical waves of compression and relaxation through a medium; air in the case of audible words.

Now, this becomes interesting, because the most modern theories on the origin of the universe hypothesize that sound waves shaped the entire universe, and they are probably still exerting their effects. Alasdair Wilkins, in the following article, writes about the concepts of dark matter and dark energy:

> "Just 30,000 years after the Big Bang, the universe started singing. Vast sound waves rang out and expanded through the primordial cosmos, their ripples determining the universe's large-scale structure. And this all fits perfectly with one particularly theory of dark energy. These acoustic waves were formed just 30,000 years after the Big Bang, as regular matter started collapsing around dense dark matter.
>
> The resultant pressure forged these waves, which oscillated outwards for about 350,000 years, tracing out the future structure of the universe as they went. By the

time the universe had cooled enough to stall these waves, matter had clumped around the center and edges of the wave, causing more galaxies to form in these areas than elsewhere."[54]

The remains of the sounds of the primeval universe are well characterized, and our entire universe is permeated by this low-frequency sound wave. On his website, John G. Cramer, Professor of Physics at the University of Washington in Seattle, writes:

"There are now two Sounds of the Big Bang items on this site, the original version produced in 2003 using the data on the cosmic microwave background from NASA's WMAP satellite mission, and a new version produced in 2013 using the data on the cosmic microwave background from the European Space Agency's Planck satellite mission. The Planck analysis has superior errors and angular resolution and goes three times as high in angular frequency".[55]

Therefore, we may not be wrong in stating that these sounds not only gave the universe the shape that we know, but that they unavoidably influenced the shape of life as well. In fact, life is part of this universe, and if sound waves shaped the universe as a whole, they must have shaped DNA-based life as well.

---

54. http://io9.com/5898846/dark-energy-confirmed-how-ancient-sound-wavesshaped-the-entire-universe

55. http://faculty.washington.edu/jcramer/BBSound.html

ULTRASONOGRAPHY

As mentioned in the introduction, I specialize in radiology with particular competence in ultrasonography, the medical imaging technique that utilizes ultrasounds to produce images of the organs in the human bodies so that we can study the morphological and structural alterations that occur during diseases.

Ultrasounds are nothing more than sound waves and, more specifically, oscillating sound pressure waves with a frequency greater than the upper limit of the human hearing range. Ultrasound simply refers to having a higher frequency.

In ultrasonography, ultrasounds are emitted by a probe. They travel through human tissues and bounce back toward the probe, reminiscent of the properties of audible echoes (hence the synonymous term "echography"). The variations in the frequency and amplitude between the emitted and received ultrasound signals are then converted in a scale of grays, and the images of the organs are formed on the screen for the radiologist to interpret.

THE PRINCIPLE OF HEISENBERG

I have been performing a number of exams with ultrasounds, and I have always been reflecting on the principle of Heisenberg as applied to ultrasounds. As it is well known, the Heisenberg principle states that the very act of performing an observation perturbs, *i.e.* changes the object that is observed. This happens because observation implies the use of some form of energy that interacts with the object that is being observed. In my case, I was thinking at ultrasounds, a form of mechanical energy; they were interacting with living human tissues under my eyes and, although they are considered absolutely safe, I wondered how this interaction could have affected the cellular and molecular structures of the organs that were being hit by these mechanical waves.

These reflections, together with the observation by physicists that sound waves (identical in physical nature to ultrasounds) shaped the universe and hence our lives, led me to go deeper into this field of research, and I began to write up findings for these research projects while still at the University of Firenze. My research was directed at two objectives: the effects of the ultrasounds at the level of DNA and the effects of ultrasounds on the brain and the functioning of the mind.

There exists very scarce literature on the effects of ultrasounds at the level of DNA, and this is quite odd given the universality of sound waves and their role in shaping the universe since the Big Bang. A very recent paper published by researchers at the Department of Radiological Sciences of the University of Toyama in Japan demonstrated that certain sequences of bases in DNA respond to ultrasounds.[56]

The following are subtitles of a broader report on observational studies on the use of ultra sound with prostated cancer cells.

Regulation of gene expression in human prostate cancer cells with artificially constructed promoters that are activated in response to ultrasound stimulation.[57]

---

56. Ultrason Sonochem. 2013 Jan;20(1):460-7. doi: 10.1016/j. ultsonch.2012.05.007. Epub 2012 May 24.

57. Ogawa R, Morii A, Watanabe A, Cui ZG, Kagiya G, Kondo T, Doi N, Feril LB Jr.

> **NOTE:** This is a continuation of the research studies outlined above.

These researchers demonstrated that there are sequences of bases in DNA, called "promoters" that are activated by ultrasounds. You can compare this phenomenon to a remote control; you can open the doors of your car with a metal key or, in modern cars, you can use a remote control that opens the doors without touching the lock. However, even if the radio wave from the car remote control does not touch the car, the energy emitted by the remote control actually physically interacts with the receiver that, in turn, opens the door. We have always known that genes can be activated by "touching" them with chemical molecules, designated transcriptional factors. Now, thanks to the work of the Japanese scientists, we realize that genes can also be activated with sound waves (in this case ultrasounds) without "touching" them.

Please consider that this is an extremely revolutionary concept that has not yet caught the attention of biologists and medical doctors. In fact, the entire *corpus* of molecular biology, pharmacology and medicine is based on the concept that genes are activated only by transcriptional factors that physically interact with them ("touch" them), and all drugs are designated with this (now limited) concept in mind.

If we further elaborate this concept, we may understand the enormity of this discovery, an enormity that probably was not even realized by the researchers from Japan themselves: let's make the example of masculinizing hormones such as testosterone (feminizing hormones could be used as an example as well). At puberty, testosterone causes effects such as deepening of voice, growth of chest hair, growth of Adam's apple, and more.

All of these effects are due to the fact that testosterone, a steroid hormone, interacts with its receptor that is a protein, and the complex testosterone/receptor physically attaches to the DNA and activates all the genes that cause the biological effects reported above.

AMAZING DISCOVERY

Now think if all the effects of testosterone, but also those of feminizing hormones, of steroids, of vitamins D and A, of thyroid hormones (they all work in the same manner: activating genes by attaching to DNA) could be obtained, stimulated, inhibited, and modulated by the claps of the hands or by the sound of a voice or, more realistically, by an ultrasound-generating device (we shall see later that we actually do not need mechanical or electronic devices to generate ultrasounds; vocal organs suffice). We could switch on and off genes at will, from a distance, without the need of drugs, pills or injections. And, unlike conventional pharmacology, we could switch on and off the genes of other people with or without their consent, and we could do this on several people at the same time. And why limit this to people? We could do this on animals and plants, bacteria and viru es. Now that we have broken the code, we could use ultrasounds to modify the functions of all forms of life without even touching them.

To put this in other terms: if we know the sequences of DNA that respond to ultrasounds (and we now know them), we could modulate the ultrasounds (an extremely easy task) to take control over the entire genetic information of the biosphere.

I fully realize that the potential is enormous and that it can be used for good or for evil purposes. Here, I prefer to concentrate on the "good" aspects of this extraordinary discovery that saw my research group at the forefront together with researchers from the University of Arizona.

PUBLISHED STUDY ON EFFECTS OF ULTRASOUNDS ON MENTAL STATES

On May 29th, 2012, and on June 1st, 2012, almost at the same time, Hameroff *et al.* and our research group published two independent studies demonstrating the effects of diagnostic ultrasounds on mental states.[58]

Here it has to be remembered that the information in all three of our brains is ultimately the information at the level of the DNA. In the case of the first brain, the one inside our heads, the human DNA codes for the shape and functions of neurons and glial cells. Hameroff and colleagues working at the Department of Anesthesiology of the University of Arizona in Tucson demonstrated that the same

---

58. Brain Stimul. 2013 May; 6(3):409-15. doi: 10.1016/j.brs.2012.05.002. Epub 2012 May 29. Transcranial ultrasound (TUS) effects on mental states: a pilot study. Hameroff S1, Trakas M, Duffield C, Annabi E, Gerace MB, Boyle P, Lucas A, Amos Q, Buadu A, Badal JJ. J IiME. 6 (1): 23-28, 2012. Transcranial sonography in the diagnosis, follow-up and treatment of Myalgic Encephalomyelitis/Chronic Fatigue Syndrome. Ruggiero M , Fiore MG, Magherini S, Esposito S, Morucci G, Gulisano M Pacini, S.

ultrasounds that are routinely used to visualize our organs improved subjective mood compared to a placebo and showed safe neurophysiological effects on brain function that could be used for modulating conscious and unconscious mental states and disorders. According to their hypothesis, ultrasounds act via intra-neuronal microtubules, which apparently resonate in the same megahertz range. A few weeks after the publication of this article, Hameroff, based on these and other observations, wrote a seminal paper listed in PubMed that poses a fundamental line of thought: "How quantum brain biology can rescue conscious free will."[59]

CHRONIC FATIGUE SYNDROME AND ULTRASOUND OBSERVATIONS

At about the same time, we were studying the effects of ultrasounds on a mysterious disease, Myalgic Encephalomyelitis, also designated (improperly) Chronic Fatigue Syndrome (ME/CFS). This complex disease involves the brain, the immune system and the gut. It is clear now that this disease may be nothing else than a disease of the "forgotten" organ: the microbiome. In those days of 2012, however, we still were analyzing one organ at the time, and we were focusing our attention on the effects of the ultrasounds on the first brain with the goal of finding a quick fix for the painful symptoms that affect patients with ME/CFS.

---

59. Front Integr Neurosci. 2012 Oct 12;6:93. doi: 10.3389/fnint.2012.00093. eCollection 2012. Hameroff S.

In our study, we merged a neural biofeedback with the effects of the ultrasounds on brain functions and we observed that heart rate significantly decreased from 81 beats per minute (bpm) at the beginning of the procedure to 71 bpm at the end of the procedure, and to 70 bpm 10 minutes after the end of the procedure. Conversely, systolic blood pressure increased from 115 mm/Hg (10 minutes before the procedure) to 125 mm/Hg (10 minutes after the end of the procedure). This observation was important in the context of ME/CFS, because cardiovascular symptoms and hypotension are common in ME/CFS patients, and it has been suggested that hypotension associated with orthostatic stress may impair neurocognitive functioning in ME/ CFS patients with postural tachycardia syndrome. We thought that the observed increase in systolic blood pressure in the absence of a concomitant increase in heart rate or diastolic pressure was of particular significance for ME/CFS, and we interpreted these findings as if ultrasound stimulation of the brain was associated with increased cardiac output.

This, in turn, could alleviate the most common symptoms reported in ME/CFS: shortness of breath, dyspnea on effort, rapid heartbeat, chest pain, fainting, orthostatic dizziness and coldness of feet. In addition, we found out that application of ultrasounds to the brain together with neural biofeedback increased muscle strength when the biceps muscle was voluntarily contracted. Considering that the lack of muscle strength is one of the major symptoms of ME/CFS (the noun "fatigue" is not casual), we thought that this observation might have been relevant.

During our studies on the effects of the ultrasounds on mental states, we observed that the US Military, and more precisely the Defense Advanced Research Project Agency (DARPA), was studying prototypes of ultrasound devices aimed at improving mental abilities, reducing stress and improving overall brain performances. In an article published in 2010, Justin Barad described the work of Dr. William J. Tyler, who posted on the blog of the Department of Defense "Armed with Science" his work on Transcranial pulsed ultrasound stimulation of the brain.

According to Barad, Dr. Tyler described his research as follows:

> "Through a recent grant made by the Defense Advanced Research Projects Agency (DARPA) Young Faculty Award Program, our research will begin undergoing the next phases of research and development aimed towards engineering future applications using this neurotechnology for our country's warfighters. Here, we will continue exploring the influence of ultrasound on brain function and begin using transducer phased arrays to examine the influence of focused ultrasound on intact brain circuits".[60]

More recently, the University of Queensland in Australia reported that ultrasounds could help patients with Alzheimer's to recover their memory and their overall mental faculties. In the following article from this most recent observation (March 2015), it is thus described:

---

60. http://www.medgadget.com/2010/09/darpa_funding_transcranial_pulsed_ultrasound_to_stimulate_soldiers_brains.html

"Queensland scientists have found that non-invasive ultrasound technology can be used to treat Alzheimer's disease and restore memory. University of Queensland researchers discovered that the innovative drug-free approach breaks apart the neurotoxic amyloid plaques that result in memory loss and cognitive decline. ...
"With an ageing population placing an increasing burden on the health system, an important factor is cost, and other potential drug treatments using antibodies will be expensive," Professor Götz said. "In contrast, this method uses relatively inexpensive ultrasound and microbubble technology which is non-invasive and appears highly effective".[61]

SOUND MAY CHANGE THE WORKING OF OUR GENES

Here, our prediction made in 2012 is confirmed; ultrasound can be used (from remote) *in lieu* of chemical drugs (in this case antibodies) that have to physically "touch" the cell machinery.

At this point, we may conclude that research institutions from all over the world (from Arizona to Italy, from Japan to Australia, not to mention the Pentagon) all agree that the sound (and by extension, the word) can change the working of our genes and, if directed toward the genes and the cells of our first brain, the working of our mind. When I mention the word "word", one may think that I am exaggerating, because ultrasounds are one thing, the sound waves of

---

61. http://www.uq.edu.au/news/article/2015/03/alzheimer's-breakthrough-uses-ultrasound-technology.

the primeval universe another thing, and audible sounds (with actual words among those) are a different thing.

Nothing could be more wrong, not only because all types of sounds, including ultrasounds, are essentially the same physical phenomenon. In actuality, there are ultrasounds all around us, natural ultrasounds emitted by all types of animals to communicate and, therefore, to influence gene expression at all levels.

In 2004, Narins and collaborators working at the University of California, Los Angeles wrote:

> "Several groups of mammals such as bats, dolphins and whales are known to produce ultrasonic signals which are used for navigation and hunting by means of echolocation, as well as for communication. In contrast, frogs and birds produce sounds during night- and day-time hours that are audible to humans; their sounds are so pervasive that together with those of insects, they are considered the primary sounds of nature. Here we show that an Old World frog (Amolops tormotus) and an oscine songbird (Abroscopus bogularis) living near noisy streams reliably produce acoustic signals that contain prominent ultrasonic harmonics. Our findings provide the first evidence that anurans and passerines are capable of generating tonal ultrasonic call components and should stimulate the quest for additional ultrasonic species."[62]

---

62. J. Acoust. Soc. Am. 115 (2), February 2004.

Here it is important to highlight the words "their sounds are so pervasive that together with those of insects, they are considered the primary sounds of nature". In other words, it is now proven that ultrasounds are also among the primary sounds of nature!

And what about the rodents that are so close to us in terms of genetic evolution? In 1975, Laurence H. Roberts published an article in the *Journal of Zoology* entitled "Evidence for the laryngeal source of ultrasonic and audible cries of rodents" reporting that:

> "The audible cries of three species of young myomorph rodents were found to be emitted through the nose and the mouth, buccal and nasal cavity resonances being involved in the production of the formant structures of the emitted cries. Ultrasonic cries were found to be emitted mainly through the mouth, with no evidence for the involvement of cavity resonances. Nerve sectioning experiments on adult and young rats implicated the larynx as the source of both their audible and their ultrasonic cries. However, consideration of the considerable differences in physical structure between the typically "vocal" audible cries and the ultrasonic cries, as well as other differences noted in the experimental conditions here and elsewhere, leads to the conclusion that the rodent larynx may operate in two quite different sound production modes."[63]

---

63. Volume 175, Issue 2, pages 243–257

The "words" of animals around us contain ultrasounds that quite possibly influence gene expression and the functioning of the brain. It is interesting to notice that even though we, as humans, cannot hear ultrasounds (and this is the very reason for their denomination), nevertheless, we are equipped to respond to them, albeit in an indirect way (and without the need for a machine). In fact, in 1997, Henry demonstrated that:

> "Vertebrates are able to perceive the pitch of a series of harmonics, even when the fundamental frequency has been removed from the acoustic stimulus. Neural periodicity responses corresponding to the "missing fundamental" frequency of sonic stimuli have been observed in the auditory system of several animal species, including our own."

THE RELATIONSHIP BETWEEN THE MICROBIOME AND ULTRASOUNDS.

At this point, only one element is missing to have a coherent picture of how "the word" shaped and is shaping the universe and our lives as well. The still missing concept that I am to develop now is the relation between ultrasounds and the microbiome.

MANY MICROBES ARE FRIENDLY

Until recently, "microbes" were considered bad things and synonymous with infectious disease. With the discovery of the microbiome, we are beginning to shift this paradigm and now write of "our microbial friends". We are learning that the microbiome and humans constitute a complex and dynamic, ever-changing ecosystem, and we are adapting our thinking to this new concept. Some prejudice against microbes still exists, but we shall not be swayed by this when we study the next paper recently published in Trends Mol Med. (2014 Jul;20(7):363-7) and entitled "Sounding the death knell for microbes?". Here, the authors, who work at the School of Forensic and Investigative Science of the University of Central Lancashire in the UK, demonstrated that ultrasounds can kill bacteria and, therefore, they postulate that ultrasounds could be used as antibacterial agents devoid of all the side effects of, for example, antibiotics.

This study corroborates the principle that ultrasounds can perform the task of drugs without their side effects and presumably at a much less expensive cost (with some dismay for pharmaceutical industries). But this study also demonstrates, as if it were necessary, that ultrasounds do actually influence microbial behavior. And it could not possibly have been different. Life on this earth began with unicellular organisms, a sort of primordial bacteria, and remained unicellular until recently. Therefore, the sound waves that shaped the universe and the DNA must have shaped microbes much earlier than multicellular organisms.

Now comes the difficult part from the technical point of view: how can we use the ultrasounds to modulate or to rebalance the function of an organ that is so dispersed as the microbiome? In other words, it is easy to direct the ultrasound waves toward the brain, and we published a seminal work describing this technique 's influence on autism.[64]

But how can we target an organ that has no anatomical seat? Essentially, first I had to find the microbial species constituting the healthy core human microbiome, and this had already been done; then I had to isolate their DNA, an easy task for any laboratory, with particular reference to those sequences that respond to ultrasounds and that had been identified by the Japanese radiologists in 2012. Then, I had to collect the ultrasound signature from those DNAs, just as is normally done with a conventional diagnostic ultrasound system. The final step was to reverberate this signal into the solution merged with the ultrasound waves that resonate in the range of biological ultra structures as demonstrated by Hameroff et al.

At that point, I had the microbiome immersed in the sound waves of the universe, i.e. the most perfect form of symbiosis between the human and non-human parts of ourselves. We are certainly encouraged by our initial observations. Please be aware that we need to do a lot more research, and we are doing that. It is our goal to perfect and enhance the effects that we have already observed and publish them as soon as the further research is completed. We are excited about the positive, effective use of ultrasonography in conjunction with our work with the microbiome to improve the quality of all of our lives.

---

64. *Front Hum Neurosci.* 2014 Jan 15;7:934. *A New Methodology of Viewing Extra-Axial Fluid and Cortical Abnormalities in Children with Autism via Transcranial Ultrasonography.* Bradstreet JJ, Pacini S, Ruggiero M.

12

An Introduction to the History and the Future of Immunotherapy

The importance of immunotherapy is finally being re-introduced as a prominent tool in the arena of proactive and preventative strategies used to fight anything that can threaten the overall health and wellness of human beings. When used in conjunction with treatments like chemotherapy and procedures like radiation, immunotherapy collaborates with these modern medicine techniques and helps pack a one-two punch against viruses and diseases like we have yet to see. The impact of using 21st century medical technologies and medicines, along with aiding and boosting the body's own internal combative systems designed to stave off disease, makes perfect sense.

So why did it take so long to come back to this forgotten theory? If the body consists of all of its own integrated systems, functions and self-regulating features, why would we assume that, given the proper fuel and maintenance, this perfect machine could not fight off any medical threats? In short, immunotherapy is a practice based off the premise that if we can supply the body with exactly what it needs and sanction the immune system to work in harmony with the body, not only will disease pose much less of a threat, but if problems do occur, the immune system should be strong enough to combat any army of viruses or diseases, especially in conjunction with modern medicine and its practices.

The formal definition of immunotherapy is: "A treatment of disease by inducing, enhancing, or suppressing an immune response. Immunotherapies designed to elicit or amplify an immune response are classified as activation immunotherapies, while immunotherapies that reduce or suppress are classified as suppression immunotherapies" (Wikipedia). What we really see from this definition is that there are actually two different immunotherapeutic approaches. Activation immunotherapy and suppression immunotherapy play a critical role in the different circumstances of the individual being treated.

Much as it sounds, activation immunotherapy is used to stimulate and intensify the natural power of the immune system. We see the use of activation immunotherapy in conjunction with other medical techniques and medicines to boost the immune system to help increase the chances of both rejecting and destroying tumors in the body. Since the late 1980s, activation immunotherapy has played a role in the fight against cancer and, specifically, malignant tumors.

It sounds counterintuitive to introduce a toxin into the body. After all, we are trying to live healthy lives. When the Father of Immunology, William Coley began his career in fighting cancer, he injected bodies with different forms of Streptococcus. By doing so, he cured many from their terminal conditions. When we inject what is now known as "Coley Toxins" into a subject, their immune system kicks into high gear, and in many cases, is able to use that infection to fight the cancer. It makes sense that 99% of the time, we would want to be strengthening and assisting the body in building the strongest immune system possible. In fact, why would one ever really want to decrease their immunity? Upon initial evaluation, you would think adding bacterial toxins into a system would only open up a world of problems and create illness. Coley proved many times that there was a critical need to activate the immune system in order to free the subject from cancer. This method was not perfect, as it did not work for all, and many of his subjects did die from the addition of the live bacteria.

It would only make sense that decimating one's immune system would open up a world of problems. Although rare, there is a very real and critical need for some to decimate their immune system; in most cases it is only for as short a period of time as needed. This would be classified as suppression immunotherapy. According to Wikipedia, "Immune suppression dampens an abnormal immune response in autoimmune diseases or reduces a normal immune-system response to prevent rejection of transplanted organs or cells." Yes, immune suppression is something that most people will never have deal with, but it can play as critical a role in some as enhancing immunity does in most.

THE FATHER OF IMMUNOTHERAPY DR. WILLIAM COLEY

Although immunotherapy was used in ancient times and documented briefly in the 13th century, Dr. William Coley was considered the Father of Immunotherapy as he used those historic documentations to propel his research on immunotherapy for cancer. Coley was born in Westfield, Connecticut in 1862 and spent his professional career split between being a surgeon and a researcher, with his main focus on cancer. Coley discovered that by provoking the immune system with bacteria, in some cases there were positive results based on the response of, or boost in the immune system. This discovery helped crown Dr. Coley as the pioneer of cancer immunotherapy.

Dr. William Coley's fascination with cancer and immunotherapy grew with his curiosity about how something considered bad (bacteria) could ultimately help the larger picture (cancer). Coley's curiosity regarding cancer immunotherapy peaked after losing a patient to bone cancer. Searching through old medical records, Coley came across a case of peculiar interest. The records told the story of a man that had been diagnosed with sarcoma. Coley noticed that during his fight with sarcoma, the patient had suffered through an infection and dangerously high fever. The information that blew Coley away was the fact that after the patient fought off the fever and infection, his tumor had disappeared.

Coley continued to scour hospital records for any cases similar to that initial one he found. During his research, he found a few other cases with very similar results and tracked down several like-minded physicians who were putting the same pieces to this puzzle together. It was then that Coley theorized that by provoking a response from the immune system due to post-surgical infections that patients would fare better when dealing with cancer. This began years of trial and error on Coley's behalf, but it ultimately set everything in motion for the benefits of immunotherapy on a large scale. Dr. William Bradley Coley passed away in April of 1936, but the work he started over 100 years ago piqued the interest of another up-and-coming doctor and researcher, Dr. Marco Ruggiero.

DR. RUGGIERO DISCOVERS DR. WILLIAM COLEY'S WORK

Over the past 30 years, Dr. Ruggiero has been a prominent player in bringing the importance of immunotherapy back to the forefront of the medical world. Dr. Coley's original theories and findings on immunotherapy established a foundation, which led Dr. Ruggiero to rediscover Coley's original views that strengthening the immune system would help fight disease almost a century after Dr. Coley died. When William Coley began his work 100 years ago, genetics and DNA had yet to be discovered, and very little was known about the immune system. Dr. Coley had stumbled on the effectiveness of fighting cancer and disease by stimulating the immune system almost by mistake. Knowing only a small fraction of what we know today regarding medicine, biology, anatomy, the immune system and the general inner workings of the human body; Dr. Coley was hot on the trail of major medical breakthroughs regarding immunotherapy. Coley's work and theories were not kept secret or classified by Coley in any way; in fact, Dr. Coley was so intrigued with his findings that he sought out some of the best doctors and researchers from around the globe to help build his case.

42 PROMINENT SCIENTISTS VALIDATED DR. COLEY'S WORK

More than 42 prominent scientists on both sides of the Atlantic Ocean validated Dr. Coley's observations on the importance of a strong immune system, and these were some of the most highly regarded medical scientists in the world at the time.

DR. COLEY'S WORK DISAPPEARS FOR 50 YEARS

For reasons unknown, Dr. Coley's findings all but disappeared for over 50 years. Sometime in the 1960s, the databases at both the National Library of Medicine as well as the NIH unearthed articles discussing immunotherapy from both Czech and German sources. Today, you can use the medical search engine, "PubMed" to find these articles from the 60s.

DR. RUGGIERO BECOMES A WORLD LEADER IN IMMUNOTHERAPY

The importance of this story is not the way in which Dr. Ruggiero stumbled across Dr. William Coley's research from 100 years earlier. What really mattered was what Marco saw in these early studies that focused on the importance of a strong immune system and its role in almost every aspect of healthy living. Rather than summarizing the fascinating stories of how Dr. Ruggiero began to put all the puzzle pieces of immunotherapies and how it can do everything from stave off disease to manage the body to self heal, here, in his own words, are transcripts of Dr. Ruggiero sharing his history of how he became a leading authority on immunotherapy.

In 1990, I was a young researcher, a practicing doctor, and working as a visiting scientist at the National Cancer Institute of the NIH in Bethesda, MD. We were working on macrophages.

Macrophages are a type of white blood cell that ingests foreign material. They are key players in the immune response to foreign invaders of the body, such as infectious microorganisms.

Normally, they are found in the spleen, connective tissues and liver of the body. They also circulate in the bloodstream and, when they circulate, they are called monocytes.

In those days, the hottest topics in cancer biology were the so-called "oncogenes", those genes in our DNA that, once mutated, cause the onset of cancer, its progression, and its metastasis. One of these oncogenes was known to regulate the function of macrophages and it was involved in a variety of human cancers.

The oncogene that was the object of our research is called the human c-fms oncogene, and it is a gene coding for a protein that regulates the function of macrophages; this protein is aptly called "macrophage colony-stimulating factor".

We published this paper in the Proceedings of the National Academy of Science of the USA, which is probably the most prestigious non-commercial publication in science.

We were working on the human c-fms oncogene. We published this paper in the *Proceedings of the National Academy of Science* of the USA, which is probably the most prestigious non-commercial publication in science.

DR. RUGGIERO PUBLISHES SCIENTIFIC PAPER ON MACROPHAGE ACTIVATING FACTOR

About four years later, a scientist published a paper about a protein that he called *the macrophage activating factor*, rather than the *stimulating* factor. He further described the effects of macrophage activation as a rare rat-borne disease called osteoporosis. We combined our research in time to publish these results at the 18th World AIDS Conference in Vienna, Austria.

So, what is this protein on which we were working in the 90s. It was, of course, the GcMAF. Even though it can be used as support in conjunction with conventional medical procedures, it cannot be defined as a drug because it is a protein that we all have in our body. It is often produced during an immune response. We can liken this protein to insulin, or vitamin D. Insulin is a hormone and Vitamin D is not a vitamin at all; it is a hormone produced by our skin when it is irradiated by ultraviolet radiation.

Now, what do we know about this protein 25-27 years after its discovery and characterization? We know that this protein does many more things in addition to stimulating macrophages. We now know that it is essential for the development and function of the immune system, as well as of the brain and the central nervous system. It is also essential for immune surveillance.

IN 2014 A NEW DISCOVERY IS MADE

About one year ago, working in our laboratories in the UK and Italy, we made a further observation. That is, this protein in our body does not circulate alone as a pure protein. It is always physiologically associated with a fatty acid, which is called oleic acid. From this discovery, we developed a molecule, which actually resembles the assembly of GcMAF in our bodies.

We then were able to successfully develop types of food that have different definitions (you can call them probiotics), which naturally contain this type of molecule, among many other things. Now, why do we need this molecule to be used in conjunction with established medical treatments and protocols with different conditions?

Because just like when you develop diabetes, when your body is unable to produce enough insulin, or you develop rickets or osteoporosis and you are not able to produce enough vitamin D, there are many conditions when the body is unable to produce sufficient quantities of oleic acid, GcMAF. Therefore, it seemed rational to provide this molecule from the outside, until a year ago, when we realized that GcMAF is not in our body alone, but it is always associated with other molecules and until we developed these foods containing these natural molecules.

And now, we are developing a full range of possibilities, and we can administer GcMAF as an edible product to everyone. This food containing GcMAF is not just for those with health challenges and compromised immune systems, but maybe just as importantly functions as a major support of the immune system for all of us blessed with good health. We are using it as a preventative interventional technology to help our immune system function at a high level. This is a great strategy that all of us should consider as part of a quality-of-life system.

We are developing food that is naturally rich in GcMAF. Therefore, we can now say that 120, 130 years ago, after the first observations of William Coley, we are now truly entering a new era of immunotherapy. By the way, it was at the end of 2013 when, in the magazine *Science*, cancer immunotherapy was heralded as the breakthrough of the year; let's remember that it is not such a novel concept.

> **NOTE:** This food we are developing and using is not a replacement for established medical treatments, drugs or protocols. This food is not a cure or treatment for any disease. It is, in fact, a support working in conjunction with recognized and established medical treatments and procedures. It is important that you always consult with your health professional or allopathic physician when embarking on any nutritional program. In no way is this to be construed or conveyed as a treatment for diseases. It acts by supporting the immune system, and that is simply a good support strategy when used in conjunction with standard medical practices

VITAMIN D RECEPTOR

VDR stands for "Vitamin D Receptor." Now, you may wonder, what does vitamin D have to do with all this? Well, the point is that GcMAF, when it is associated with oleic acid, is part of a nutritional pathway, which is the vitamin D axis. We published this in a peer-reviewed journal a few years ago. Because of this, we can think of GcMAF as a nutritional component. When investigated further, it is a nutritional component of our metabolism, in which we may see deficiencies.

So there are conditions in which deficiency of GcMAF is responsible for a number of symptoms.

Now, because of this, when last year we described the molecular assembly and these novel functions of GcMAF, we published this paper of ours in a journal that is called *Nutrients*. As you probably know, scientific articles are ranked according to the impact they have on the medical-scientific community. There are sort of "hit parades", so to speak, and one bibliometric index that is used to measure the quality and quantity of attention that a given article receives in the medical-scientific community.

It is called the AltMetric. As of today, AltMetric has tracked millions of scientific articles published in peer-reviewed journals. When I say "millions," I mean articles that led to discoveries that in turn led to the award of Nobel Prizes. Well, this article of ours, where we describe this novel role of GcMAF, is ranking in the top five percent. This means that it is receiving a great deal of attention by the scientific and medical community because of the potential of this observation of ours, and also because we are beginning to realize that it is not a drug, it is not a hormone, it is not a cytokine interleukin. It is a nutritional component of which we may be severely deficient.

We have learned that most anti-cancer strategies can be greatly assisted with the integration of a proper nutritional plan. When I say a proper nutritional plan, I mean essentially a very low-carb, very high protein, and very high anti-inflammatory fat daily consumption. When I say *no carbs*, I mean no more than 15% of the daily caloric intake needs to come from complex carbohydrates. with a series of tricks and strategies in order to avoid insulin peaks. 50-55% of the daily caloric intake has to consist of proteins, preferably of vegetable origins, and the fats have to be anti-inflammatory fats like extra virgin olive oil, coconut oil, and flaxseed oil.

When I say immune anti-cancer surveillance, I mean to empower the immune system with molecules that are able to stimulate the immune system, just like oleic acid and GcMAF. When I talk about the healthy, uncorrupted, human core microbiome, the third brain, I am referring to this relatively new organ of ours that Dr. Ruggiero revealed earlier in his "Eureka moment", which actually is not new at all. It is new because until three or four years ago, no one knew about it.

Three or four years ago, we knew that we had gut microflora, but we thought they were just there living peacefully with in us. Three or four years ago, it was discovered that our human cells are out-numbered by microbial cells ten-fold. But even more interesting is that we have known since 1953, when Watson and Crick discovered that the genes actually reside in the DNA, that life can be defined as genetic information that replicates itself. If we look at our human life, which means our human genes, we have about 22,000 genes. We can say that the instructions to make a human are contained in about 22,000 genes. But if we look at our cells, considering now all of the microbes that are part of our microbiome, or Microbiota, you find out that we have eight million genes (The Microbiome Project by NIH).

We can say that from the genetic point of view, from the point of view of genetic information, we are less than 1% human, because more than 99% of the genetic information that is in the body right now is due to microbes that participate in this virtual organ that is dispersed throughout the gut as well as several places within the body. This virtual organ, which participates in the metabolism of the body, is as essential as the liver and all the other organs of the body. Now, we know that the microbiome is essential for the development of the human brain as well as the development of the human immune system. Therefore, if we want to deal with the immune system, we cannot disregard the microbiome. Supplying the microbiome with genetic information is very important in the success of immunotherapy.

NUTRITION IS THE FOUNDATION OF A QUALITY OF LIFE SYSTEMIC APPROACH TO LIFE

We have discovered that the role of nutrition is not only beneficial in improving the quality of life for some incurable cancer patients, but it also helps to support (as we have published in our observational studies) the effects of whatever cancer treatment comes to mind: from the conventional radiation therapy and chemotherapy as well as more novel approaches. In addition, as we demonstrated in our previously published peer reviewed paper, it has also been shown to reduce the side effects of chemotherapy in some people.

I must add that this protocol of ours has not shown any side effect after 11,000 people have been treated. It has also been effectively used as a complementary support to conventional therapies like radiotherapy, chemotherapy or whatever is necessary.

Why? The answer is simple. Radiotherapy and chemotherapy have known side effects, which are mainly imputable to the killing effects on rapidly dividing cells, like those of the GI tract or the killing effects on the microbiome. With this protocol of ours, you support the healthy immune system on a daily basis. You provide a lining for the entire gut, due to the adhesion molecules present in this super food, so in many cases you significantly decrease the side effects of chemotherapy.

We have observed cases where some young girls, who were subjected to chemotherapy in the morning, were able to have dinner at a restaurant with friends the same evening. Again, this was during chemotherapy. So you see, the primary role of the flexibility of a natural approach to cancer is to support common conventional treatment. This tells you about the potential and the flexibility of a natural, immunotherapeutic approach to cancer. And when I say "immunotherapeutic approach", I do not refer only to a direct support in conjunction with recognized cancer treatments and their effect on cancer, but also on some side effects.

CANCER CAN FOOL OUR IMMUNE SYSTEM

If our immune system would not be fooled by the cancer cells, cancer simply would not exist, because our immune system is very well equipped to recognize cancer cells and to kill them right away. From a statistical point of view, we have had cancer cells in our body since the very moment we are born. We keep accumulating cancer cells throughout our lives, but most of the time. our immune system is able to recognize these cancer cells as foreign enemy cells and to kill them—that is, to induce their physiological death, which is called apoptosis. But cancer cells also follow the rules of evolution; otherwise we would not have cancer at all. At some point in time, they become disguised as cancer cells. It is like an enemy is invading our country, but they do not wear the uniform that makes us recognize them. They wear our uniforms. So we do not recognize them as enemies, and they are able to perpetrate their crimes. Now, this is where our approach, called immunotherapy, has been observed in our published papers to have protective effects by supporting the immune system.

MACROPHAGES AND OTHER CELLS OF OUR IMMUNE SYSTEM

Our published observations focus on empowering the macrophages and other cells of the immune system with the ability and the tools to recognize even those cancer cells that are disguised as normal cells. It is as if we are giving our soldiers scanners so that they can scan all the cells and identify those that are enemies, even if they don't look like it at first. So the immunotherapy approach involves empowering the immune system and giving back to it the ability to discover, attack, and kill the cancer cells. That's why it's so different from the traditional approach of chemotherapy. Chemotherapy is like throwing bombs. They kill everything, the bad and the good, and sometimes more the good than the bad. But the immunotherapeutic approach is extremely targeted, because we're not killing the cancer cells, we're letting the immune system kill the cancer cells.

NOTE: Macrophage stimulation (immune system support) is not a treatment for any disease or illness. It is simple a way to stimulate and support a healthy immune system in the quest to ward off diseases. This is not a cure for any disease of illness. It is a preventative approach to empower the immune system to get the support it needs to potentially ward off attacks to it. Our whole approach with our patients is to add safe and scientifically validated natural protocols (like immune system support) on top of conventional medical treatments to do everything possible to improve the quality of life for all of our patients.

As we have stated over and over, these natural super foods we have discovered and produced are not a substitute for proven medical treatments, drugs and protocols. These super foods are not drugs, and in no way should the reader think this is some miraculous cure to disease or illness. It is, again, to do everything we can to supply the body with the best nutrition possible for it and most importantly, for our three brains. This strategy of support for the immune system is an approach that certainly requires more study.

IMMUNOTHERAPY IN CONJUNCTION WITH CONVENTIONAL MEDICAL PROCEDURES

In my opinion, you can integrate immunotherapy in association or in combination with any regimen that you are using today. This immunotherapeutic approach can also be adjusted according to individual cases. I will give you an example of what we do in our clinic. First, we implement a very strict ketogenic detoxifying diet. When I say detox, I say that we open an entire area of discussion. So we adopt these integrated approaches of a ketogenic detox in combination with the super foods we created. We have patients that do this while they are undergoing radiation or chemotherapy, and the effect so far has been synergistic with the two approaches. Let's just call them the old conventional and the new immunotherapeutic, they are not antagonistic. They do not fight each other. They are synergistic, so that the combined effect is more than the addition of the two approaches taken singularly.

We have been on this path now for years. By complementing the body and boosting its own immunities, we have seen success in regards to one's overall health. Aside from disease, this is a way of living that will only improve your overall chances of staying healthy and living longer. I cannot neglect the impact of TDOS Syndrome in the realm of immunotherapy. There is no doubt that those four co-factors, (Toxicity, Nutritional Deficiency, Overweightness, Stress) play a huge part in the big picture. I became familiar with TDOS Syndrome just a year ago, when I had the honor and privilege to meet Peter Greenlaw, at the Autism One meeting. I fully subscribe to his point of view, even though at the time, we didn't know the details of the TDOS Syndrome and Solutions. I had been following and applying nutritional solutions, and naively, without knowing the details. we have witnessed positive results, since 2010 or 2011.

We conducted a study in 2010, well before I met Peter. In the study, we had three groups of stage IV cancer patients that we observed in a hospital near Florence, Italy. We had about thirty patients in each group. All these patients were diagnosed with stage IV cancer, metastatic, and they had all done whatever they could; conventional and complementary approaches. We are talking about surgery, radiation therapy, and chemotherapy, everything you can think of. Essentially, they were sent home to put their things in order and to prepare to die because there was nothing else they could do.

So at that point, we intervened and essentially observed that the three groups had some absolutely identical features, but they differed in something that was really important, which was nutritional deficiency and the proper balance of mineral elements and proteins. Now, according to this division based on nutrition, the three groups had a prognosis of six months to four years. We began working on just the nutrition part, correcting the deficiencies and reducing an excess of fat cells as well as working to fix what we call futile cycles.

We conducted this study without any drugs, we simply worked on nutritional balance and detoxification with plenty of water (2-3 liters of water per day), and we were able to shift the prognosis from six months to four years. And I'm talking about Stage four terminal cancer patients. This was published in a peer-reviewed medical journal, *The American Journal of Immunology*, in 2012. Obviously, when we approach a patient with immunotherapeutic strategies, we implement this nutritional approach.

But I wanted to relate this story just to say that I fully agree with an approach that is based on dense nutrition that includes nutrients, vitamins and wide array of minerals. If you do not correct nutritional deficiencies, if you do not fix protein imbalances, if you do not get rid of the bad fat that is accumulating toxins, then every therapeutic approach, whether conventional or unconventional, will have a diminished chance of success.

The foundation of immunotherapy is simple: use the greatest tool we have to fight off all diseases, viruses, etc. That tool is the human body. This is why all of Dr. Ruggiero's work flows so well within "The New Health Conversation".

DR. RUGGIERO TALKS ABOUT THE FACT THAT OUR BODY IS THE MIRACLE

The miracles are not in any one product or protocol; the miracle is the human body itself. Our job is to find cutting-edge resources to fuel and boost the body's natural defense systems. The dessert cup is a nutritional technology, thirty years in the making by Dr. Ruggiero, his wife Dr. Stefania Pacini and his colleagues, and their pioneering research into nutritional science and microbiology.

Bovine milk, colostrum and 40 strains of bacteria are what make up the super food, which is capable of reconstituting genetic information for the third brain. Essentially, that means that Dr. Ruggiero discovered a way to support your immune system on a daily basis. By strengthening the immune system, following Dr. Ruggiero's protocols, and integrating nutritional solutions (dense nutrition), we have a much greater shot at living healthier longer.

Our mission in this book was not only to educate you about these monumental discoveries, but to share ways to strengthen your microbiome. In the next several years, we hope to see a shift in the importance of the microbiome on a global scale. It can be argued that a healthy microbiome is as important as a healthy first brain. In the future, we may see a shift toward the primary care of our second and third brains, as we now know this care is as important as the care we give to our first brain. We cannot thank Dr. Marco Ruggiero for his tireless efforts in the lab and at the bedside, and his unwavering curiosity to explore unchartered territories. After 30 years of work, we are on the verge of rediscovering the human body as the miracle that it is.

CONCLUSION

Your Third Brain is Part of "The New Health Conversation" Series

The mission of "The New Health Conversation"™ is to make you aware of what is available. This includes making you aware of the totality of the problems we face, and most importantly offering you multifaceted solutions to deal with the problems we have made painfully apparent to you.

We made you aware that not only do we have a brain in our heads, but we have a second brain in our GI tract. Then, we showed you the interconnection between these two brains and the important role they play in our emotional quality of life.

We highlighted that there are specific foods that will allow for the first brain and second brain to function at their highest potential. We have further introduced you to the understanding of the title of this book, *Your Third Brain*, the amazing "Eureka Moment" for Dr. Ruggiero that led to the impact of this epiphany as to what it could mean for mankind if there was a way to interact with this "Third Brain".

For most scientists, just identifying the impact of this newfound organ might have been worthy of a potential Nobel Prize. For Dr. Ruggiero, this realization simply opened up more pathways for research and discovery. Knowing that this third brain, created at birth, is nourished by genetic information – the genetic information contained in the foods we consume – is an extraordinary and uncommon concept for even the most versed clinician.

With that in mind, Dr. Ruggiero and his colleagues discovered that the third brain was genetic information that was created at birth, and contained eight million Genes. This discovery occurred when they identified that the combination of colostrum and mothers' breast milk, along with 40 bacteria, fungi yeast, and microbes, formed the microbiome. After hundreds of attempts, they were able to create a food that contained the genetic information of the microbiome.

The genetic information contained in this super food, created by Drs. Ruggiero and Pacini, is food for the third brain. This naturally created super food contains the genetic information for the microbiome, and has been named the "Microbiome Protocol". This is the foundational strategy for a higher quality of life.

Equally as important is the Microbiome Regimen. Dr. Ruggiero and colleagues combined the Microbiome Protocol, along with The Microbiome Regimen, utilizing very specific nutritional technologies. They have stated multiple times that The Microbiome Protocol and The Microbiome Regimen are inseparable. You can have the best genetic information provided by the super food for the microbiome, but if your gut flora is not properly fed utilizing the Microbiome Regimen, then the Microbiome Protocol will not be as effective.

It is the synergistic relationship of the protocol and regimen, which Dr. Ruggiero and his team consume daily, that makes them truly effective. This combination yields the best preventative interventional strategy.

As we have pointed out, a vibrant immune system plays a critical role in surveillance against invaders that potentially harm our quality of life. We encourage everyone to embrace and use The Microbiome Protocol in conjunction with The Microbiome Protocol Regimen. They should always be used in synchronicity, and they are never mutually exclusive. This is the secret to a higher quality of life, which has now been demonstrated and experienced by many people.

We invite you to join us in the potential for a much higher quality of life for you and your community. Drs. Ruggiero and Pacini, and their colleagues, have worked tirelessly for years to bring this gift of scientific knowledge and discovery to the world. Their solutions allow us the opportunity to have the most robust and effective immune system, should we choose to follow their protocols.

Their whole goal has been to use their discoveries for maximizing our quality of life, our wellness potential and our ability to live healthier longer. The discoveries uncovered in *Your Third Brain* are for the vast majority of our readers who are blessed with good health and who want to maximize their wellness potential.

We hope this book is also valuable to medical professionals who thirst to become aware of the scientific observations made by Dr. Ruggiero and his team. We believe that professionals who are willing to step outside the box and use the Microbiome Regimen and Protocol, in addition to more recognized and established medical protocols, can improve the quality of life for their patients.

Remember, the impossible is only impossible until it is possible. Now that you know, what will you do?

Peter Greenlaw, 2015

AUTHOR'S NOTE: These discoveries are in no way a replacement for established and proven medical treatments—instead, they have been used in combination with allopathic physicians and health professionals. Our goal has been to improve the quality of life for people who are facing medical challenges, and just as importantly, for healthy individuals who want to prolong their healthy lifestyles utilizing these quality-of-life solutions.

APPENDIX

PAPERS ON GLUCOSE METABOLISM AND HUMAN DISEASES

Pacini S, Aterini S, Salvadori M, Ippolito E, Ruggiero M, Amato M. "Cellular proliferation and second messenger formation altered by dialysis membranes." *Nephrol Dial Transplant.* 1997 Mar;12(3):500-4. PMID: 9075131 [PubMed - indexed for MEDLINE] Free Article

Casamassima F, Pacini S, Dragotto A, Anichini M, Chiarugi V, Ruggiero M. "Intracellular diacylglycerol: a mitogenic second messenger proposable as marker of transformation in squamous cell carcinoma of the lung." *Lung Cancer.* 1996 Sep;15(2):161-70. PMID: 8882982 [PubMed - indexed for MEDLINE]

Pacini S, Ruggiero M, Casamassima F, Santucci MA, Milano F, Ranaldi F, Vanni S, Giachetti E. "Study of second messenger levels and of sugar catabolism enzyme activities in transformed cells resistant to ionizing radiations." *Biochem Mol Biol Int.* 1995 Sep;37(1):81-8. PMID: 8653091 [PubMed - indexed for MEDLINE]

Aterini S, Ippolito E, Salvadori M, Pacini S, Ruggiero M, Amato M. "Second messenger formation altered by different dialysis membranes in human leukocytes." *Kidney Int.* 1994 Aug;46(2):461-6. PMID: 7967358 [PubMed - indexed for MEDLINE]

Del Rosso M, Anichini E, Pedersen N, Blasi F, Fibbi G, Pucci M, Ruggiero M. "Urokinase-urokinase receptor interaction: non-mitogenic signal transduction in human epidermal cells." *Biochem Biophys Res Commun.* 1993 Jan 29;190(2):347-52. PMID: 8381273 [PubMed - indexed for MEDLINE]

Ruggiero M, Casamassima F, Magnelli L, Pacini S, Pierce JH, Greenberger JS, Chiarugi VP. "Mitogenic signal transduction: a common target for oncogenes that induce resistance to ionizing radiations." *Biochem Biophys Res Commun.* 1992 Mar 16;183(2):652-8. PMID: 1550572 [PubMed - indexed for MEDLINE]

Ruggiero M, Wang LM, Pierce JH. "Mitogenic signal transduction in normal and transformed 32D hematopoietic cells." *FEBS Lett.* 1991 Oct 21;291(2):203-7. PMID: 1936266 [PubMed - indexed for MEDLINE] Free Article

Chiarugi V, Basi G, Quattrone A, Micheletti R, Ruggiero M. "The old and the new in transformed cell signalling: glycolysis, diacylglycerol and protein kinase C." *Second Messengers Phosphoproteins.* 1990;13(1):69-85. Review. No abstract available. PMID: 2286934 [PubMed - indexed for MEDLINE]

Chiarugi V, Bruni P, Pasquali F, Magnelli L, Basi G, Ruggiero M, Farnararo M. "Synthesis of diacylglycerol de novo is responsible for permanent activation and down-regulation of protein kinase C in transformed cells." *Biochem Biophys Res Commun.* 1989 Oct 31;164(2):816-23. PMID: 2684158 [PubMed - indexed for MEDLINE]

Chiarugi VP, Magnelli L, Pasquali F, Basi G, Ruggiero M. "Signal transduction in EJ-H-ras-transformed cells: de novo synthesis of diacylglycerol and subversion of agonist-stimulated inositol lipid metabolism." *FEBS Lett.* 1989 Jul 31;252(1-2):129-34. PMID: 2668028 [PubMed - indexed for MEDLINE] Free Article

Ruggiero M, Srivastava SK, Fleming TP, Ron D, Eva A. "NIH3T3 fibroblasts transformed by the dbl oncogene show altered expression of bradykinin receptors: effect on inositol lipid turnover." *Oncogene.* 1989 Jun;4(6):767-71. PMID: 2543945 [PubMed - indexed for MEDLINE]

Ruggiero M, Lapetina EG. "Sustained proteolysis is required for human platelet activation by thrombin." *Thromb Res.* 1986 Apr 15;42(2):247-55. PMID: 3715802 [PubMed - indexed for MEDLINE]

Ruggiero M, Lapetina EG. "Leupeptin selectively inhibits human platelet responses induced by thrombin and trypsin; a role for proteolytic activation of phospholipase C." *Biochem Biophys Res Commun.* 1985 Sep 30;131(3):1198-205. PMID: 4052085 [PubMed - indexed for MEDLINE]

Made in the USA
Middletown, DE
05 September 2017